Zeineb Teyeb
Mariem Essouri
Naziha Khammassi

Urinary tract infection in women: How is it treated?

Zeineb Teyeb
Mariem Essouri
Naziha Khammassi

Urinary tract infection in women: How is it treated?

Imprint
Any brand names and product names mentioned in this book are subject to trademark, brand or patent protection and are trademarks or registered trademarks of their respective holders. The use of brand names, product names, common names, trade names, product descriptions etc. even without a particular marking in this work is in no way to be construed to mean that such names may be regarded as unrestricted in respect of trademark and brand protection legislation and could thus be used by anyone.

Cover image: www.ingimage.com

This book is a translation from the original published under ISBN 978-620-6-72486-5.

Publisher:
Sciencia Scripts
is a trademark of
Dodo Books Indian Ocean Ltd. and OmniScriptum S.R.L publishing group

120 High Road, East Finchley, London, N2 9ED, United Kingdom
Str. Armeneasca 28/1, office 1, Chisinau MD-2012, Republic of Moldova, Europe
Printed at: see last page
ISBN: 978-620-6-74001-8

Contents

1 Introduction

Urinary tract infection (UTI) is a medical condition in which pathogenic microorganisms, most commonly bacteria, are present in the urinary system[1]. The urinary system includes the bladder, ureters, urethra and kidneys[2]. UTIs can manifest themselves in several ways, depending on the site affected. Clinical manifestations range from simple burning of the micturition to septic shock. Urinary tract infection is the second most common community infection after respiratory tract infection, with a worldwide incidence of 404.61 million in 2019 [3].

This common condition affects women in particular, because the female anatomy bacterial access to the urinary tract[4]. In fact, around 10% of women have at least one episode of UTI per year, and 60% have at least one episode of UTI in their lifetime[5].

There are several types of urinary tract infection in women: cystitis, pyelonephritis and urethritis. The clinical picture varies with age and gender, and can be misleading and aspecific in older subjects[6]. The use of bacteriological and radiological investigation makes diagnosis and consequently therapeutic management much easier, even in the presence of an isolated fever.

Antibiotic treatment is obviously still the cornerstone of therapeutic management, and the prognosis is vital.

Urinary tract infection (UTI) is still a topical issue, especially in view of the increasingly alarming level of antibiotic resistance in a country ranked as the 2nd largest consumer antibiotics in the world[7,8].

The management of antibiotic resistance requires close collaboration between healthcare professionals and health authorities, as well as raising awareness in the medical community [9, 10].

Hence the importance studying the evolutionary profile of female urinary tract infections as a function of clinical form, bacteriological profile and therapeutic strategy in Tunisia.

2 Objective

The main aim of our study was to describe the therapeutic management of UTIs in women outside pregnancy in an internal medicine department.

The secondary objective was establish the clinical, biological and bacteriological characteristics of UTIs in women outside pregnancy in an internal medicine department.

1. Type and duration of study

We conducted a retrospective, descriptive, monocentric study of patients hospitalized for UTI at the Internal Medicine Department of the Razi Hospital in Tunis between January 2016 and August 2023.

Urinary tract infections are defined as :

Acute cystitis: defined as inflammation of the bladder wall secondary to a bacterial agent. It is manifested by burning of the micturition, pollakiuria, dysuria, urgency and hypogastric pain.

Acute pyelonephritis (AP): defined as bacterial infection of the renal parenchyma and renal collecting system. It is manifested, in association with signs of cystitis, by fever and chills, and/or lower back pain, often unilateral and/or sometimes digestive signs.

Other definitions :

Anemia: Hemoglobin < 12g/l

An antibiotic susceptibility test is a laboratory test used assess the sensitivity of germs to different antibiotics.

CRP high if above 10mg/L

Septic DCI: sepsis with hypotension (PAS<90 mmHg or 30% fall from baseline resistant to vascular filling).

ESBL risk factors: hospitalisation within 6 months, antibiotic therapy (Amox, C2G, C3G, FQ) within 6 months and history of ESBL colonisation or UTI within 6 months.

Fever: temperature above or equal to 38.5°C

HyperAlpha1globin:> 3.5g/l, Hyperalpha2globin:>8.5g/l

Hyperleukocytosis: white blood cell count > 1000/^L 0, Leukopenia: white blood cell count<4000/^L

Hyperpolynucleosis: polynuclear count > 7000/^L , Neutropenia: polynuclear count< 1500/^L

Hypotension: BP<= 90/60

Renal failure if creatinine clearance<60 mm/min (MDRD)

Lymphocytosis: lymphocyte count >4000/iiL, Lymphopenia: lymphocyte count<1500/^L

Significant leukocyturia if urine leukocytes >= 10^4 EB /ml

Procalcitonin positive above 0.5 ng/ml

Quick SOFA (qSOFA): 2 of the 3 following factors are positive: Respiratory rate>=22, SGC<15/confusion/Disorientation, PAS<=100 mmHg

Sepsis: if q SOFA>=2

Biological inflammatory syndrome: elevation of the VS >20 mmH1, CRP>10 mg/l, alpha 1globulin > 3.5g/l and alpha 2 globulin>8.5g/l

Improvement in SIB: reduction in CRP and SV of 50% or more.

Thrombocytosis: Platelet count <400000/^L,

Thrombocytopenia: platelet count <150000/^L

VS raised above 20 mm H1

2. Population studied

2.1 Inclusion :

We chose include female patients, hospitalized in the Internal Medicine Department of Razi Hospital, aged over 15 years, who had a urinary tract infection between January 2016 and August 2023.

2.2 Non-inclusion criteria :

The male gender

Age < 15 years

Non-bacterial UTI

Asymptomatic bacteriuria

Pregnant woman

2.3 Exclusion criteria :

Incomplete file

ECBU not available

2.4 Collection and processing of files :

We collected information from the medical records of hospitalized patients over 15 years of age. included age, medical history, immunosuppressant use, habits, clinical characteristics, physical examination, bacteriological and radiological findings, severity criteria (quickSOFA (qSOFA)), treatment and course.

3. Statistical analysis :

Data collection and statistical analysis were carried out using IBM SPSS Statistics version 26. The categorical variables are presented as counts and percentages. Variables following a normal distribution were expressed as mean +/- standard deviation P .

For variables that do not follow a normal distribution, values have been presented using the median followed by the interquartile range.

4. Bibliography :

The search was carried out using the google search engine, PubMed, Science direct, HAL open science via the words: urinary tract infection/ infection urinaire, antibiotic resistance/ antibioresistance, SPILF and STPI.

5. Conflict of interest :

No conflicts of interest have been declared.

1. Descriptive study

1.1 Epidemiological data

Between January 2016 and August 2023, 62 patients were included in our study. The average annual incidence was 7 cases.

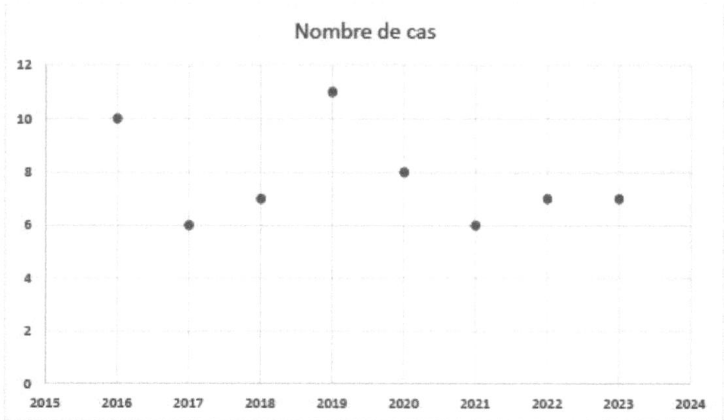

Figure 1 : Distribution of patients year of hospitalisation

1.2 Age

The mean age of the patients was 59.31±17.64 years (17-92 years):

-Forty-two per cent of the population were aged over 65

-Twenty-one per cent were aged 75 and over.

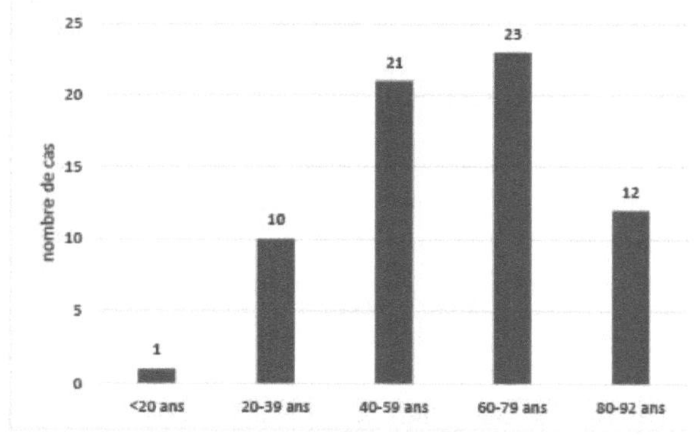

Figure 2 : Age of patients

1.3 Background

All the patients were being treated for a medical condition.

The most common antecedents were diabetes (59%) and hypertension (51%).

None of the patients included in the study had neoplasia (cancer) or AIDS.

The various antecedents are shown in Table I.

6

Table I: Medical history of patients included in the study

ATCD	Workforce	Percentage
Diabetes	37	59%
Arterial hypertension	32	51%
Dyslipidemia	31	50%
Complications of diabetes	24	39%
Chronic renal failure	23	37%
Immunodepression	23	37%
Diabetic nephropathy	9	14%
Severe renal failure	9	14%
Cerebrovascular accident	9	14%
Coronary artery disease	6	9%

Table II summarises the various autoimmune pathologies in patients in 37% of cases.

Table II: Patients' various systemic diseases

Sjogren's syndrome	9	14%
Systemic lupus erythematosus	5	8%
Multiple sclerosis	3	5%
Vasculitis	2	3%
Rheumatoid arthritis	1	1%
Inflammatory myopathy	1	1%
Systemic scleroderma	1	1%
Sarcoidosis	1	1%

Patients were receiving immunosuppressive treatment in 12% of cases.
Corticosteroids were used in 21% of patients, with a median dose of 162.86 mg (5-1000).
Figure 3 shows the different immunosuppressive drugs taken by patients.

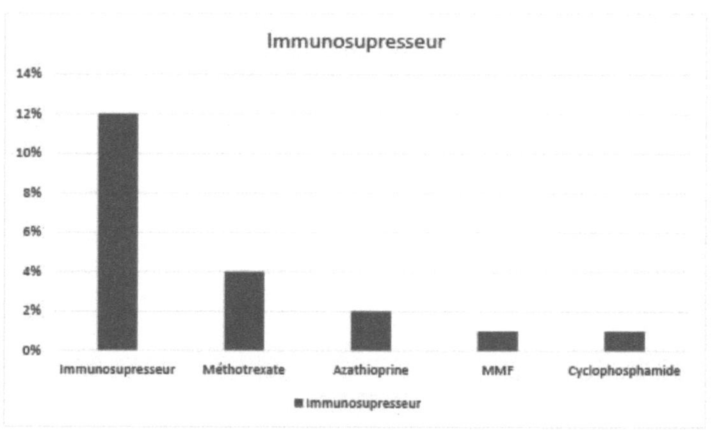

Figure 3: Use of immunosuppressants

1.4 Habits

12% of patients were smokers.

1.5 Risk factors for the carriage of multi-resistant bacteria (MRB) :

BMR risk factors included the presence of a history BMR urinary tract infection in 19% of cases, antibiotic use (fluoroquinolone (FQ), amoxicillin-clavulanic acid, Cephalosporin $2_®{}^{me}$ generation (C2G) and Cephalosporin $3^{c}{}_{me}$ generation (C3G)) and/or hospitalisation in the 6 months preceding the infectious episode in 12% and 27% of cases respectively.

1.6 Characteristics of the infectious episode

Sixty percent had acute cystitis, while 40% had acute pyelonephritis.

Table III summarises the various functional signs reported by patients.

Table HI: Breakdown of functional signs of UTI

	Workforce	Percentage
Burning while urinating	20	32%
Dysuria	19	30%
Fever	16	25%
Lower back pain	15	24%
Imperiositis mictionalis	11	17%
Urinary leakage	9	14%
Pollakiuria	8	13%
Suprapubic pain	6	9%
Macroscopic hematuria	5	8%
Acute urinary retention	2	3%
Nausees	2	3%
Vomiting	2	3%

1.6.1 Cystitis: 37 cases included

1.6.1.1 Functional signs :

- Urinary burning was reported by 32% of patients.
- Dysuria was present in 24% of cases.
- Imperiosity of micturition was present in 19% of patients.
- Urinary leakage was present in 13% of patients.
- Pollakiuria was present in 11% of cases.
- Hematuria was present in 8% of patients.

1.6.1.2 Physical examination :

- The mean temperature measured was 36.9°C (standard deviation = 0.34), with extremes ranging from 36° to 37.5°C.
- Sensitivity to lumbar shaking was absent in all patients.
- No sepsis was observed.

1.6.1.3 Imaging :

Of the 10 ultrasound scans performed when cystitis was diagnosed, showed any abnormality suggestive of an upper UTI.

1.6.1.4 Biology :

Blood count

All patients had a complete blood count (CBC).

Haemoglobin ranged from 6.3 g/dl to 14.2 g/dl. Anemia was observed in 59.4% of cases.

Platelet counts ranged from 55,000/^L to 460,000/^L. Thrombocytopenia was noted in 5.4% of cases and thrombocytosis in 2.7%.

The white blood cell count ranged from 4200/^L to 348000/^L. Hyperleukocytosis was present in 16.21%. of the patients had leukopenia.

Neutrophil counts ranged from 1940/LIL to 29440/LIL. Neutrophilic polynucleosis was present in 19%. There was no objective neutropenia.

Lymphocytes ranged from 650/lL to 3380/lL. Lymphopenia was present in 24.3% of cases. However, there was no objective lymphocytosis.

Markers of inflammation :

Biological inflammatory syndrome was absent in all patients.

Kidney function :

The average creatin value measured was 99.16, with extremes ranging from 47 to 576.

The mean clearance value measured was 72.78, with extremes ranging from 6.17 to 127.90.

Renal failure was present in 13.5% of cases.

Functional renal failure was present in 10.8% of cases.

One patient had chronic renal failure associated with a

1.6.1.5 Cytology:

All patients underwent a cytobacteriological examination of their urine.

The mean leukocyturia in the patients was 526×10^3 with extremes ranging from 12×10^3 to 9000×10^3. Ninety-one percent of cases had leukocyturia. Leukocyturia was absent in 3 patients.

Mean hematuria was 43×10^3 with extremes ranging from 0 to 200×10^3. Two patients had microscopic hematuria (5.4%).

1.6.1.6 Culture :

culture isolated 6 germs. The most frequent Escherichia coli (E. coli), followed by Klebsiella pneumoniae (KP) and other BGN.

Table IV summarises the different germs isolated in the culture of the patients' ECBUs.

Table IV: Different germs isolated during cystitis

Germs	Number	%
Escherichia coli	18	56%
Klebsiella pneumoniae	8	25%
Enterococcus	2	6,25%
Enterobacter cloacae	2	6,25%
Proteus mirabilis	1	3%
Staphylococcus saprophyticus	1	3%

Thirteen per cent of cases were culture negative, but cystitis was suspected in the presence of urinary symptoms with leukocyturia explained by previous antibiotic treatment.

1.6.1.7 Antibiogram and type of resistance :

Antibiotic susceptibility testing was not carried out in 5 of the cases studied, due to the absence of an isolated germ.

Among the 32 cases where antibiograms were performed :

The presence of BMR was detected in 29.7% of cases. More specifically, bacteria secreting extended-spectrum beta-lactamase (ESBL) were identified in 13.5% of cases.

Two cases of resistance to aminoglycosides have been identified, each with a distinct phenotype:

-One case with the Tobramycin-Amikacin (TA) phenotype.

-Another case with the Gentamicin-Tobramycin-Netilmicin (GTN) phenotype.

There was one case each of resistance to Macrolides, Rifampicin and Fosfomycin.

The resistance profile of the germs is shown in figure 4.

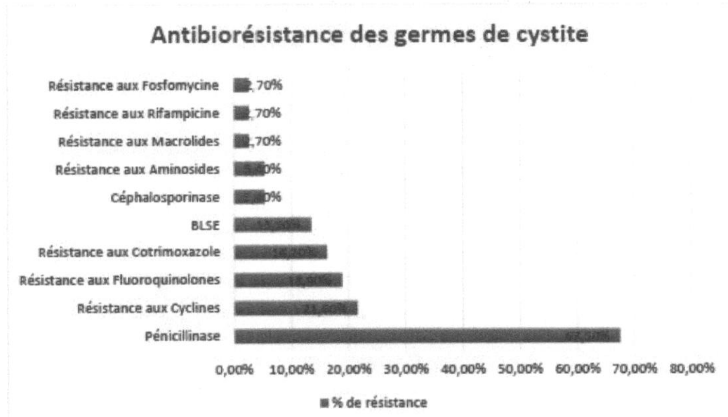

ESBL: extended spectrum beta-lactamase-secreting bacteria

Figure 4   :Antibiotic resistance of germs responsible for cystitis

The resistance profile of E. coli strains implicated in cystitis is shown in Figure 5.

Resistance profile of E. coli during cystitis

Figure 5   Antibiotic resistance profile of E. coli strains in cystitis cystitis

The resistance profile of KP strains implicated in cystitis is shown in Figure 6.

Resistance profile of Klebsiella pneumoniae during cystitis

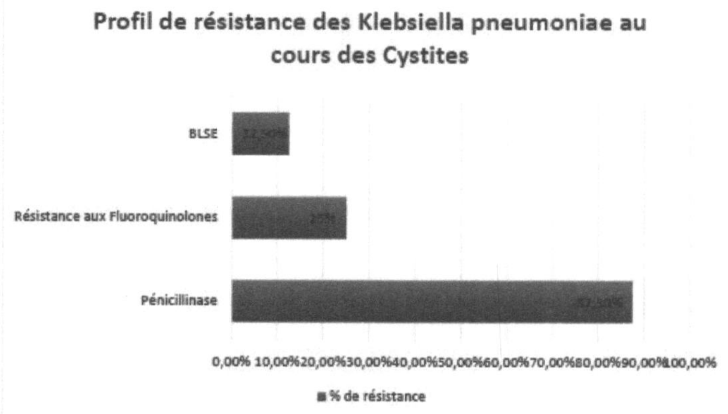

ESBL: extended spectrum beta-lactamase-secreting bacteria

Figure 6   Resistance profile of K.P. strains during cystitis

1.6.1.8 Blood culture: no blood culture was taken as there was no fever.

1.6.1.9 Treatment :

Ninety-seven per cent of patients had received antibiotic treatment.

FQ is the most frequently prescribed antibiotic.

One patient was transferred to another department before antibiotic therapy was started.

Antibiotics were administered intravenously in 13.5% of cases.

Table V shows the antibiotics prescribed.

Table V: Drugs prescribed for cystitis.

Antibiotics	N	%
Fluoroquinolone	**12**	**32,4%**
Cephalosporin	**11**	**29,7%**
Fosfomycin	6	16,2%
Cotrimoxazole	2	5,4%
Imipeneme	1	2,7%

A change of therapeutic class adapted according to the antibiogram was necessary in 3 patients.

Descalation was noted in 2 patients.

Escalation to C3G in one patient.

Table VI summarises the adaptation of antibiotic therapy following antibiotic susceptibility testing.

Table VI: New antibiotics prescribed after antibiotic susceptibility testing

Antibiotherapy	Number of cases
Cotrimoxazole	1
Ciprofloxacin	1

Cephalosporin	1	

The average duration was 4.93 days, with a maximum of 7 days and a minimum of 1 day (when Fosfomycin was taken).

1.6.1.10 Evolution :

Clinical and biological improvement was achieved within the first 48 hours of antibiotic initiation in 86.1% of cases.

A follow-up ECBU was positive in three patients (table VII).

Table VII: Germs isolated at follow-up ECBU tests

Germs	Resistance	Numbers
E. coli	Sensitive	1
Klebsiella pneumonia	Multi-resistant bacteria	2

Recurrence within the first 6 months was observed in 3 cases.

Of these, 2 patients had a multi-resistant germ: E. coli (N=1) and Proteus mirabilis (N=1).

1.6.2 Acute pyelonephritis: 25 cases included

1.6.2.1 Functional signs :

- Lower back pain was felt by 48% of cases.
- Suprapubic pain was noted in 12% of cases.
- Hematuria was observed in 8% of cases.
- Acute urinary retention[1] was observed in only one case.
- Digestive disorders were noted in 3 cases (12%).

1.6.2.2 Physical examination :

- Temperature data collected on admission, prior to administration of the antibiotics, showed a range of variation from 36 to 39.5 degrees Celsius, with an average of 37.23°C. Fever was present in 28% of cases.
- The physical examination revealed sensitivity to lumbar strain in 32% of cases.
- A patient presented with urinary retention complicating a bladder globe.
- A qSOFA (Quick SOFA) calculated at 2 was objective in 2 patients and calculated at 3 in 3 patients.
- Three patients were found to have sepsis and two to be in septic shock.

1.6.2.3 Renal imaging :

Ultrasound was prescribed in 64% of cases. Sixteen percent of patients had ultrasound abnormalities. These findings included :

- 2 cases of nephritis,
- 1 case of non-obstructive kidney stones
- 1 case of urinary distension upstream of a bladder globe with ureteritis

which required emergency drainage.

uroscan was performed or prescribed.

1.6.2.4 Biology :

<u>Blood count :</u>

All patients had a blood count:

Haemoglobin ranged from 3.6 g/dl to 14.7 g/dl, with a mean of 10.7 g/dl. Seventy-two percent of patients had anemia.

Platelet counts ranged from 49,000/^L to 604,000/^L. Twelve percent of patients had thrombocytopenia. Thrombocytosis was present in 0.08% of cases.

The white blood cell count ranged from 1,050/^L to 28,150/^L, with a mean of 9869/LIL. Hyperleukocytosis was present in 28% of cases and leukopenia in 12%.

Polynuclear neutrophils (PNN) ranged from 890/lL to 20,120/lL, with a mean of 7060/lL. Neutrophilic polynucleosis was present in 28% of cases and neutropenia in 0.04%.

Lymphocytes ranged from 590/lL to 6330/lL, with a mean of 1851/lL. Lymphopenia was present in 36% of cases and lymphocytosis in 0.04%.

<u>Inflammatory parameters :</u>

A biological inflammatory syndrome was present in 96% of cases.

One patient had an elevated CRP without elevation of other markers

<u>CRP</u>

The mean CRP measured was 91.39 mg/l, with extremes ranging from 15 to 346 mg/l. One hundred percent of patients had an elevated CRP.

<u>VS :</u>

The mean SV measured was 71.76 mm H1 with extremes ranging from 18 to 150 mm H1. Ninety-four percent of patients had an accelerated SV.

<u>EPP :</u>

Protein electrophoresis showed hyperalphal-globulinemia and hyperalpha2-globulinemia in 76% (N=19) of cases each.

<u>Procalcitonin :</u>

The mean value was 1.16 ng/ml with a minimum value of 0.54 ng/ml and a maximum of 3 ng/ml. Procalcitonin greater than 2 ng/ml was observed in 0.08% of cases (N=2).

<u>Kidney function :</u>

The mean creatinine value measured was 114.63 lmol/l, with extremes ranging from 51 to 379 lmol/l.

The mean clearance value measured for the patients was 60.11 ml/min with extremes ranging from 11.86 to 121.39 ml/min.

Acute renal failure was observed in 44% of cases.

Chronic renal failure was present in 11 patients.

The types of renal failure are shown in table VIII.

Table VIII: Renal function during ANP

	Inf Pection	
	Number	NA Percentage
Acute renal failure (ARF)	11	44,0%
Functional	9	36,0%
Organic	7	28,0%
Obstructive	1	8,3%

1.6.2.5 Cytology :

The mean leukocyturia was 269×10^3 (standard deviation = 373) with extremes ranging from 0 to 1000×10^3. Leukocyturia was noted in 92% of patients.

Leukocyturia was absent in 8% of cases.

In our sample, the average hematuria in patients was 5×10^3, with extremes ranging from 0 to 25 x103. Microscopic hematuria was observed in 20% of cases.

1.6.2.6 Culture :

A germ was isolated in 92% of cases.

A negative culture was present in 2 patients.

Table IX shows the different germs isolated during ANPs.

Table IX: Germs isolated during pyelonephritis

Culture and germs	N	%
E. coli	13	56%
KP	4	17,3%
BGN non precise	3	13%
Proteus mirabilis	1	4,3%
Enterobacter	1	4,3%
Enterococcus faecalis	1	4,3%

E.coli: Escherichia coli, KP: Klebsiella pneumoniae, BGN: gram-negative bacilli

1.6.2.7 Antibiogram and type of resistance :

BMRs were present in 20% of cases.

ESBL bacteria were present in 8% of cases.

Penicillinase was present in 47.8% of cases.

Resistance to FQs was 34.7%.

Bacteria were susceptible in 2 cases.

The different antibiotic resistance levels of germs isolated during NAPs are shown in Figure 1.

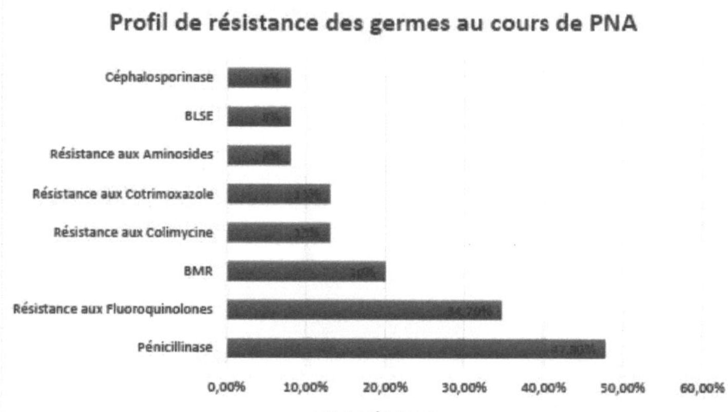

Figure 7: Resistance profile of germs during pyelonephritis

The resistance profile of E. coli strains isolated from NAPs is shown in Figure 7.

Antibiotic resistance profile of Escherichia coli strains

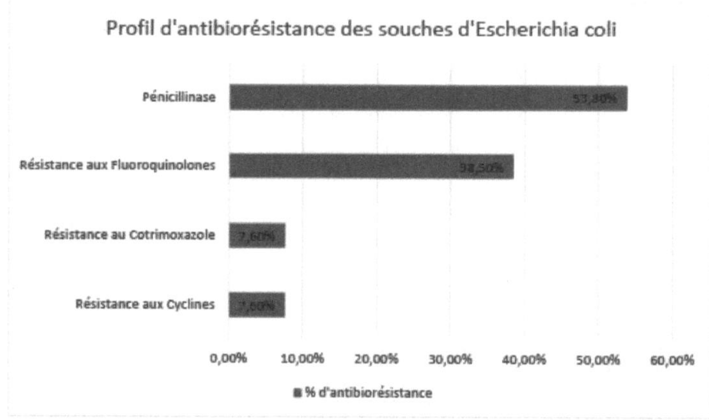

Figure 8: Escherichia coli resistance profile during pyelonephritis

Figure 9 shows the rates of resistance to the various antibiotics of the KP strains isolated during the course of the NAPs.

Resistance profile of Klebsiella pneumoniae

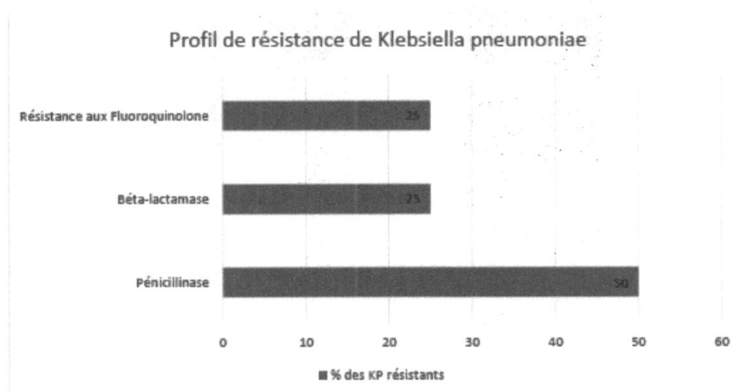

Figure 9: Resistance profile of Klebsiella pneumoniae in pyelonephritis

1.6.2.8 Blood cultures :

A blood culture was prescribed in response to the fever, with a negative culture.

1.6.2.9 Treatment :

Ninety-two per cent (N=23) of acute pyelonephritis cases in our cohort were treated with antibiotics.

Antibiotic treatment was prescribed but not given to 2 patients who had rapidly worsened clinically, requiring treatment in other departments (a medical intensive care department and a urology department).

Twenty percent of cases required treatment with C3G and gentamicin (3 cases), C3G and FQ in 1 case and C3G and metronidazole (1 case).

Table X shows the different antibiotics prescribed as first-line treatment during ANP.

Table X: Antibiotics prescribed as first-line treatment

Antibiotics	N	%
Cephalosporin 3eme generation	17	68%
Fluoroquinolone	5	20%
Aminosides	3	1,2%
Amoxicillin-Ac clavulanique	1	0,4%
Imipeneme	1	0,4%
Metronidazole	1	0,4%

A change of antibiotic according to the antibiogram was necessary in 18.8% of cases (N=3). Therapeutic escalation using imipenem in combination with an aminoglycoside was necessary in 2 patients. Fluoroquinolone therapy was de-escalated in one patient.

Table XI details the antibiotics prescribed after antibiotic susceptibility testing.

Table XI: Antibiotics prescribed after antibiotic susceptibility testing

Antibiotics	Number of cases
Imipeneme + aminoside	2
Fluoroquinolone	1

The intravenous route was necessary in 82% of cases.

Twenty patients (80%) intravenous antibiotic therapy without per os relay.

5 patients received oral antibiotics: Cefixime in 3 cases, Ciprofloxacin and Ofloxacin in 1 case each.

The average total duration of antibiotic treatment was 11.71 days, with extremes ranging from 6 to 31 days.

The average duration of use of the antibiotic relay measure is 2 days, with extremes ranging from 3 to 7 days.

1.6.2.10 Evolution :

Twenty-four percent of patients had a severe initial presentation: 2 cases of septic shock transferred to intensive care, 3 cases of sepsis (qSOFA>2) and 1 case of urinary distension on a bladder globe requiring emergency urinary drainage in a urology department.

Stable apyrexia, disappearance of back pain and urinary signs were obtained within the first 48 hours in 95.5% of cases.

An improvement in the biological inflammatory syndrome was obtained at D5 of the start of antibiotic therapy in 86.4% of patients.

Control ECBU on day 7 of TBA was negative in 12 patients.

 of the patients had an early recurrence within 6 months.

1.6.3 Particularities of UTI with BMR and ESBL:

Enterobacteriaceae were the most frequently isolated germs, in both cystitis and ANP, in 83.5% of patients. The most frequently isolated germ E. coli in 50.7% of cases, followed by KP in 19%.

Resistance to at least one antibiotic was observed in 77.6% of patients.

Taking all types of UTI together, BMR were present in more than a quarter of cases and ESBL in 13%. E.coli was the most frequent BMR and ESBL-secreting bacterium, followed by KP.

Table XXIV shows the germs isolated during all UTIs in our cohort.

Table XXIV: Different multi-resistant bacteria and bacteria secreting extended-spectrum beta-lactamase isolated during urinary tract infections

	BMR	ESBL
Total	27,4% (N=17)	12,9% (N=8)
E. coli	58,8% (N=10)	37,5% (N=3)
Klebsiella pneumoniae	11,76% (N=2)	25% (N=2)

BGN not specified	11,76% (N=2)	12,5% (N=1)
Enterobacter	5,8% (N=1)	12,5% (N=1)
Enterobacter cloacae	-	12,5% (N=1)
Enterococcus saprophiticus	5,8% (N=1)	-
Enterococcus	5,8% (N=1)	-

E.coli: Escherichia coli, GNB: gram-negative bacilli, MRB: multi-resistant bacteria, ESBL: extended-spectrum beta-lactamase-secreting bacteria.

The most frequent multi-resistance association was between betalactam and FQ at 94%, followed by betalactam and Sulfametoxazole-Trimetroprime at 52.9%, then betalactam and cyclins at 29.4%.

The association between betalactam resistance and aminoglycosides was 17.6%.

1.7 Resistance profile of E. coli :

E. coli was the germ most frequently isolated during cystitis and PNA.

Resistance to Amoxicillins was the most frequent at 64.7%, followed by Amoxicillin-clavulanic acid at 57%.

E. coli ESBL accounted for 8.8%.

Figure 10 shows the antibiotic resistance of E. coli strains isolated during cystitis and ANP.

Resistance profile of Escherichia Coli strains

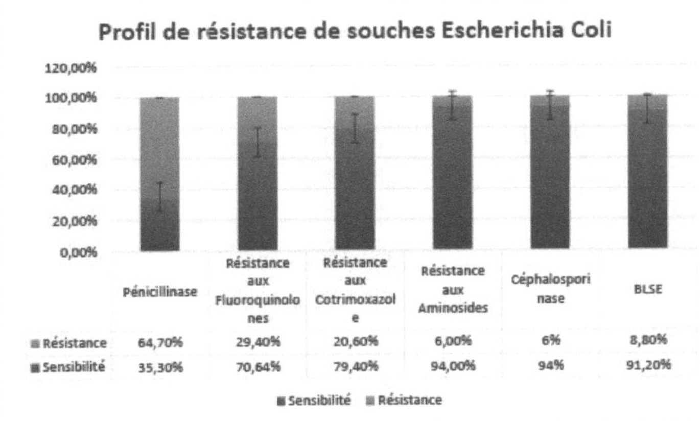

Figure 10: Antibiotic resistance of E. coli strains isolated during ANP and cystitis

1.8 Resistance profile of Klebsiella pneumoniae :

KP ranks 2nd among the most frequently isolated germs, BMR and ESBL-secreting bacteria in cystitis and PNA.

Resistance to amoxicillin and clavulanic acid was the most common, at 57.2%.

The number of secreting ESBL strains was 14.3%.

Figure 11 shows the ATB resistance profile of KP during UTIs (cystitis and PNA).

Antibiotic resistance profile of Klebsiella pneumoniae strains

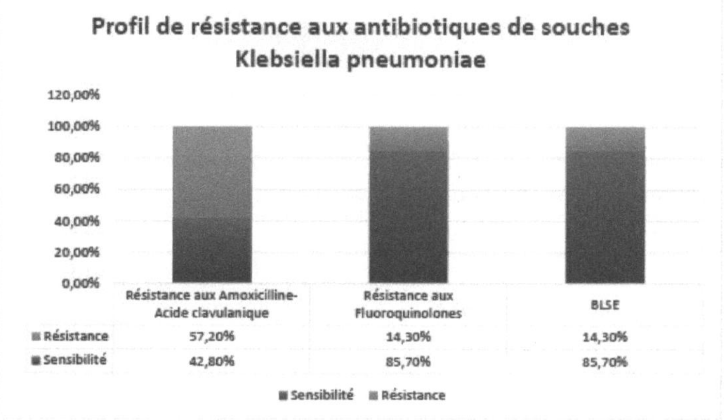

Figure 11: Antibiotic resistance of Klebsiella pneumoniae strains in pyelonephritis and cystitis.

2 Analytical study :

2.1 Association between germ resistance and terrain

2.1.1 Resistance to ATBs :

We found no statistically significant relationship between age and terrain, and antibiotic resistance.

Table IIII: Association between ATB resistance and terrain

		Resistance ATB		OR	P
		No	Yes		
Age		58,31	59,98		NS
Microalbuminuria/Proteinuria		0	1,54		NS
Arterial hypertension	No	9	19	3,079	NS
	Yes	4	26		
Diabetes	No	8	18	2,400	
	Yes	5	27		NS
Complications of diabetes	No	10	26	2,436	NS
	Yes	3	19		
Diabetic nephropathy	No	12	37	2,595	
	Yes	1	8		NS
Smoking	No	10	43	0,155	NS

		No	Yes	OR	P
	Yes	3	2		
Insufficiency renal failure chronicle	No	10	29	1,839	NS
	Yes	3	16		
Severe renal failure with CL below 30	No	11	39	1,692	NS
	Yes	1	6		
Anomalies of tree urinary	No	11	41	1,073	NS
	Yes	1	4		
Immunodepression	No	8	30	0,800	NS
	Yes	5	15		
Autoimmune diseases	No	7	28	0,708	NS
	Yes	6	17		
Immunosuppressant	No	11	40	0,688	NS
	Yes	2	5		
Corticoides	No	10	35	0,857	NS
	Yes	3	9		
History of recent urinary catheterisation	No	12	42	0,778	NS
	Yes	0	2		
Neurological bladder	No	10	42	0,159	NS
	Yes	3	2		
Intervention urological recent	No	13	41	0,627	NS
	Yes	0	2		

2.1.2 Multi-resistant bacteria :

We found a statistically significant relationship between diabetic nephropathy and bacterial resistance (p=0.013).

Patients with diabetic nephropathy are 7 times more likely to contract multi-resistant bacteria (Odds ratio =7.091).

Table XIII: Association between multi-resistant bacteria and terrain

		Bacteria multi resistant		OR	P
		No	Yes	OR	P
Age		60,55	56,88		NS
Microalbuminuria/Proteinuria		1,56	0,04		NS
Arterial hypertension	No	21	8	1,125	NS
	Yes	21	9		
Diabetes	No	22	5	2,640	NS
	Yes	20	12		

Complications of diabetes	No	28	9	1,778	NS
	Yes	14	8		
Diabetic nephropathy	No	39	11	**7,091**	NS
	Yes	3	6		
Smoking	No	37	16	0,463	NS
	Yes	5	1		
Insufficiency renal failure chronicle	No	29	11	1,217	NS
	Yes	13	6		
Severe renal failure with LC inf 30	No	36	15	0,960	NS
	Yes	5	2		
Anomalies of tree urinary	No	38	15	1,689	NS
	Yes	3	2		
Immunodepression	No	27	12	0,750	NS
	Yes	15	5		
Autoimmune diseases	No	25	11	0,802	NS
	Yes	17	6		
Immunosuppressant	No	35	17	0,673	NS
	Yes	7	0		NS
Corticoides	No	32	14	0,762	NS
	Yes	9	3		
	Yes	1	0		

2.1.3 Bacteria secreting beta lactamase :

We found a statistically significant relationship between urinary tract abnormalities and beta lactamase-secreting bacteria (p=0.016).

Patients with urinary tract anomalies are 14 times more likely to have a urinary tract infection with BLSE-secreting bacteria (Odds ratio =14.4).

Table XIV: Association between beta lactamase-secreting bacteria and terrain

		Bacteria secretante de beta lactamase			
		No	Yes	OR	P
Age		60,61	52,38		NS
Microalbuminuria/Proteinuria §		1,04	2		NS
Arterial hypertension	No	25	4	NS	NS
	Yes	26	4		

		Resistance at FQ No	Yes	OR	P
Diabetes	No	23	4	NS	NS
	Yes	28	4		
Complications of diabetes	No	32	5	NS	NS
	Yes	19	3		
Diabetic nephropathy	No	43	7	NS	NS
	Yes	8	1		
Accident vascular cerebral	No	45	6	NS	NS
	Yes	6	2		
Coronary artery disease	No	46	8	NS	NS
	IDM	5	0		
	IC	0	0		
Smoking	No	45	8	0,849	NS
	Yes	6	0		
Insufficiency renal failure chronicle	No	36	4	0,240	NS
	Yes	15	4		
Severe renal failure with CL below 30	No	43	8	0,843	NS
	Yes	7	0		
Anomalies of tree urinary	No	48	5	**14,400**	**0,016**
	Yes	2	3		
Immunodepression	No	34	5	1,200	NS
	Yes	17	3		
Autoimmune diseases	No	31	5	0,930	NS
	Yes	20	3		
Immunosuppressant	No	45	7	1,071	NS
	Yes	6	1		
Corticoides	No	41	5	2,733	NS
	Yes	9	3		

2.1.4 Fluoroquinolone (FQ) resistance:

We found a statistically significant relationship between arterial hypertension (AH) and FQ resistance (p=0.024).

Patients with hypertension had 4 times more UIL with an FQ-resistant germ (Odds ratio = 4.167).

Table IV: Association between FQ resistance and terrain

	Resistance at		OR	P
	FQ No	Yes		
Age	58,65	61,75		NS

Microalbuminuria/Proteinuria		1,40	0,50		NS
Arterial hypertension	No	25	4	**4,167**	**0,024**
	Yes	18	12		
Diabetes	No	22	5	2,305	NS
	Yes	21	11		
Complications of diabetes	No	29	8	2,071	NS
	Yes	14	8		
Diabetic nephropathy	No	38	12	0,585	NS
	Yes	5	4		
Accident vascular cerebral	No	37	14	0,159	NS
	Yes	6	2		
Coronary artery disease	No	38	16	2,033	NS
	IDM	5	0		
	IC	0	0		
Smoking	No	38	15	0,507	NS
	Yes	5	1		
Insufficiency renal failure chronicle	No	32	8	2,909	NS
	Yes	11	8		
Severe renal failure with CL below 30	No	38	13	2,192	NS
	Yes	4	3		
Anomalies of tree urinary	No	39	14	1,857	NS
	Yes	3	2		
Immunodepression	No	26	13	0,353	NS
	Yes	17	3		
Autoimmune diseases	No	24	12	0,421	NS
	Yes	19	4		
Immunosuppressant	No	36	16	0,692	NS
	Yes	7	0		
Corticoides	No	32	14	0,457	NS
	Yes	10	2		
	Yes	1	1		

FQ: Fluroquinolones

2.2 Relationship between germ resistance and prior antibiotic therapy: For the 1st episode

2.2.1 Resistance to at least one ATB :

No statistically significant relationship was found between the use antibiotics in the 6 months preceding the urinary infection and the resistance of the germs of the current infection to at least one family of ATBs.

There was no statistically significant relationship between recent hospitalisation within 6 months and the resistance of germs in the current episode of UTI.

Table XVI: Association between TBA resistance and antibiotic therapy preliminary

		Resistance No	4 ATB Yes	OR	P
History of BMR	No	11	34	3,235	NS
	Yes	1	10		
FQ within 6 months	No	12	39	1,846	NS
	Yes	1	6		
Recent hospitalisation	No	0	4	1,317	NS
	Yes	13	41		

BMR: multi-resistant bacteria, FQ: Fluoroquinolones

2.2.2 Multi-resistant bacteria :

There was no statistically significant relationship between current urinary tract infection with multi-drug resistant bacteria and previous BMR infection.

No statistically significant relationship was found between the use antibiotics or hospitalisation in the 6 months preceding the urinary infection and the resistance of the germs of the current infection.

Table XVII: Association between multi-resistant bacteria (MRB) and prior antibiotic therapy

		Resistant bacteria No	multi Yes	OR	P
History of BMR	No	35	11	2,652	NS
	Yes	6	5		
FQ within 6 months	No	37	15	0,987	NS
	Yes	5	2		
Recent hospitalisation	No	2	2	0,375	NS
	Yes	40	15		
Other Antibiotics within 6 months	No	41	15		NS
	Yes	0	0		

BMR: multi-resistant bacteria, FQ: Fluoroquinolones

2.2.3 Bacteria secreting beta lactamase :

We found a significant link between BMR antecedents and urinary tract infection with bacteria secreting extended-spectrum beta lactamase (p=0.001).

We found that patients with a history of BMR had 11.944 times more beta lactamase secrecy (Odds ratio =11.944).

Table XVIII: Association between beta lactamase-secreting bacteria and preliminary antibiotic treatment

		Beta la< No	secretante :tamase Yes	OR	P
History of BMR	No	43	3	**11,944**	**0,001**
	Yes	6	5		
FQ within 6 months	No	46	6	3,067	NS
	Yes	5	2		
Recent hospitalisation	No	4	0	1,170	NS
	Yes	47	8		
Antibiotic prophylaxis	No	49	7		NS
	Yes	0	0		

BMR: multi-resistant bacteria, FQ: Fluoroquinolones

2.2.4 Fluoroquinolone (FQ) resistance :

There was no statistically significant relationship between prior antibiotic therapy, especially fluoroquinolone therapy, and urinary tract infection with FQ-resistant bacteria in our series.

Table VIX: Association between FQ resistance and antibiotic therapy preliminary

		Resistance a to FQ No	Yes	OR	P
History of BMR	No	36	10	3	NS
	Yes	6	5		
FQ within 6 months	No	38	14	1,086	NS
	Yes	5	2		
Recent hospitalisation	No	3	1	1,125	NS
	Yes	40	15		
Antibiotic prophylaxis	No	41	15		NS
	Yes	0	0		

BMR: multi-resistant bacteria, FQ: Fluoroquinolones

2.3 Relationship between severity of infection and antibiotic resistance :

2.3.1 ATB resistance :

We found a statistically significant relationship between the type of infection (cystitis or ANP) and ATB resistance (p=0.030).

There was no statistically significant relationship between antibiotic resistance and the severity of the initial clinical presentation (sepsis or shock septic) or complications (the subsequent occurrence of septic shock, emphysematous ANP, pyonephrosis, and renal abscess) in our series.

Table XX: Association between severity infection and ATB resistance

		Resistance AГБ		OR	P
		No	Yes		
Grave	No	13	43	0,768	0,439
	Yes	0	2		
Septic shock (severe)	No	13	44	0,772	0,588
	Yes	0	1		
Guerison	No	2	5	1,418	0,698
	Yes	11	39		
Complications	No	13	43	0,768	0,439
	Yes	0	2		
Complications during treatment	No	13	44	0,772	0,588
Infection	Cystitis	6	30		**0,030**
	NAP	4	14		

ANP: acute pyelonephritis

2.3.2 FQ resistance :

There was no statistically significant relationship between severity of infection and FQ resistance.

Table XXI: Association between severity infection and FQ resistance

		FQ resistant	ince	OR	P
		No	Yes		
Grave	No	43	14	0,246	NS
	Yes	0	2		
Status of shock septic (severe)	No	43	15	0,259	NS
	Yes	0	1		
Guerison	No	6	2	1,167	NS
	Yes	36	14		
Complications	No	42	15	2,800	NS
	Yes	1	1		
Complications during treatment	No	42	16	0,724	NS
Infection	Cystitis	29	7		NS

| | | NAP | 11 | 8 | | |

ANP: acute pyelonephritis

2.3.3 Multi-resistant bacteria :

No statistically significant relationship was found between the severity of infection and urinary tract infection with multi-resistant bacteria.

Table XXII: Association between severity infection and multi resistant

		Bacteri resistai No	e multi ite Yes	OR	P
Grave	No	40	17	0,702	NS
	Yes	2	0		
Status of shock septic(severe)	No	41	17	0,707	NS
	Yes	1	0		
Guerison	No	6	2	1,167	NS
	Yes	36	14		
Complications	No	41	16	2,563	NS
	Yes	1	1		
Complications during treatment	No	42	16	0,276	NS
Infection	Cystitis	25	11		NS
	NAP	14	5		

ANP: acute pyelonephritis

2.3.4 Bacteria secreting beta lactamase :

There was no statistically significant relationship between severity of infection and ESBL UTI in our series.

Table XXIII: Association between severity infection and bacteria beta lactamase secretant

		Bacteri secretan beta lac No	e ite de tamase Yes	OR	P
Grave	No	49	8	0,860	NS
	Yes	2	0		
Status of shock septic(severe)	No	50	8	0,862	NS
	Yes	1	0		
Guerison	No	6	2	0,409	NS

	Yes	44	6		
Complications	No	49	8	0,860	NS
	Yes	2	0		
Complications during treatment	No	50	8	0,862	NS
Infection	Cystitis	31	5		NS
	NAP	16	3		

ANP: acute pyelonephritis

UI in adults is a real public health problem. It has a major impact on morbidity and mortality, with 236,790 deaths and 520,200 DALYs (Disability-Adjusted Life Years) worldwide [11]. UTIs also have a negative impact on patients' psychology and relationships, both intimate and social, leading to a reduced quality of life, particularly in women [12,13]. Because of the female anatomy, urinary tract infections (UTIs) are more common in women [14].

Diagnosis is not always straightforward. Urine culture is considered the gold standard for the diagnosis of UTIs. However, in around a third of cases, a positive culture is not obtained, and it has become increasingly clear that bacteria can be present in the healthy bladder [15].

The Enterobacteria family is predominant in UTIs with a prevalence of 89%, dominated by E. coli at 67% in a Tunisian series dating from 2019 to 2020 and 80% in a Moroccan series from 2006 to 2008 [16, 17].

We conducted a retrospective, descriptive, monocentric study of patients admitted to the Internal Medicine Department at Razi Hospital between January 2016 and August 2023.

Sixty-seven patients were included in our study. The mean age of the patients was 59 years with extremes between 17 and 93 years.

We recorded 37 cases of cystitis and 25 cases of PNA. Gram-negative bacilli were isolated in 83.58% of cases and gram-positive cocci in 7.46%. E.coli was the most frequently isolated germ at 50.7%, followed by Klebsiella pneumoniae at 20.9%. The most common medical antecedents were diabetes (55%) with complications (36%), hypertension (48%), dyslipidemia (46%), CKD (34%) and immunodepression (34%). A BMR risk factor was present in 19% of cases.

BMRs were present in 25% of cases and ESBL-secreting bacteria in 12%. The most frequently isolated BMRs and ESBLs were E.coli in 59% and 37% of cases respectively, followed by KP in 12% and 25%, other BGN and lastly gram-positive cocci (Table 10).

The most frequent association of multiple resistance was between betalactam and FQ at 94%, followed by betalactam and cotrimoxazole at 52.9%. Eleven patients (16.4%) were resistant to 3 or more antibiotic families, with maximum resistance in 6 families.

For cystitis, the most frequently prescribed probabilistic antibiotic was FQ in 32% of cases, followed by cephalosporins in 30% and Fosfomycin in 16% of cases.

Cephalosporins (C3G) were prescribed for pyelonephritis in 68% of cases, FQ in 20%, and aminoglycosides in 1.2% of cases.

According to the antibiogram, escalation of therapy was necessary in 1 case of cystitis and 2 cases of ANP.

A good clinical and biological evolution after an initial effective antibiotic treatment, or after therapeutic adjustment within the first 48 hours, was noted in 86% of cystitis cases and 95% of pyelonephritis cases.

In our series, a relationship between terrain and antibiotic resistance was found in :

- patients with diabetic nephropathy (7 times greater risk of contracting a BMR)
- patients with a urinary tract anomaly (14 times greater risk of developing a urinary tract infection with an ESBL-secreting germ).
- patients with a history of BMR infection (12 times more likely to have a secret SSBL urinary tract infection).

1. Strengths and limitations:

1.1 Type of study :

This is a retrospective, monocentric study that provides a one-off opportunity to analyse the characteristics and course of the urinary tract infection in each patient over a well-defined period of time.

However, this study is based on the collection of data from paper medical records. This exposes the study to selection bias and the risk missing information.

To better study cause and effect, we need to carry out a prospective study.

1.2 Samples :

We had access 62 records of patients hospitalised for urinary tract infection, including 37 cases of cystitis and 25 cases of pyelonephritis.

The sample is limited and subject to selection bias. The small number does not give a general idea of the bacteriological profile of urinary tract infections throughout the region. This limits the power of statistical analysis.

1.3 Hospitals :

Our study enables us assess hospital behaviour in patients urinary tract infections.

However, extrapolation to the general population becomes difficult, especially in the case of community-acquired urinary tract infections, especially given the exclusion of patients seen at outpatient clinics. Hence the non-random sample is not very representative.

1.4 Duration of the study :

A 7-year period, from 2016 to 2023, gives us a long way to go to determine exact trend.

1.5 Bacteriology :

We do not have the Minimum Inhibitory Concentration (MIC) on the antibiograms supplied by the laboratory.

2. Characteristics of urinary tract infection :

2.1 Age :

In our series, the mean age was 59 years, with extremes ranging from 17 to 92 years. The incidence of urinary tract infections was greater than 42% in patients aged over 64, with a frequency of 21% in those aged 75 and over.

It has been established that the incidence of lU increases with age, affecting 10 to 20% of people aged between 65 and 70, and 20 to 30% after the age of 80 [18].

This is explained by the menopause due to oestrogen deficiency [19], co-morbidities, the frequency of urinary incontinence affecting 38-73% of women aged over 60 [20], and the decrease in urinary Tamm-Horsfall protein levels (proteins whose role is to inhibit the multiplication and adhesion of bacteria) with age [21, 22].

2.2 Comorbidities:

Among our patients, type 2 diabetes was present in 59% and arterial hypertension in 51%. Autoimmune disease was noted in 37% of patients, with 12% on immunosuppressants and 21% on corticosteroids at the time of UTI diagnosis. Diabetes and immunodepression are considered risk factors UTIs. UTI in diabetic women is frequent, with a prevalence of 14% in a Moroccan series by El Aziz S et al and 38% in a Tunisian series by Affes et al, due to the presence of glycosuria, defective neutrophil function and increased adhesion to uroepithelial cells. [23, 24, 25].

2.3 Risk factors for multi-resistant bacteria:

The risk factors for BMR in our series include

-Antibiotics taken in the previous 6 months: 12%.

-History of UTI with BMR: 19

-Previous hospitalisation in the previous 6 months: 27%.

Studies in Tunisia (Dr Saada et al, Dr Chakroun et al) and Algeria (Dr Kalla et al) have shown a significant association between prior antibiotic therapy, invasive devices, recent hospitalisation and BMR infection[26 ,27, 28].

In an analytical study, patients with diabetic nephropathy were found to be 7 times more likely to develop multi-resistant urinary tract infections. This is explained by increased bacterial adherence facilitated by bladder hypo-contractility (autonomic neuropathy) and decreased cytokine secretion in association with glucosuria, all of which are explained by diabetes itself. A Tunisian study by Dr Saada et al , established a relationship between comorbidities including diabetes and the presence of BMR with a prevalence of diabetics of 59.4% (n = 66, IC95% : 0.50-0.68) among 111 BMR infections hospitalised from 2013 to 2019[26]. However, this was not demonstrated in an Algerian study by Dr Kalla et al [28].

These two studies found a significant association between prior antibiotic therapy, invasive devices, recent hospitalisation and BMR infection[26,28].

Urinary tract anomalies confer a 14-fold increased risk of developing an ESBL UTI and a 4-fold increased risk of developing an FQ-resistant UTI. Urinary tract anomalies are themselves a risk factor for the development of recurrent urinary tract infections, thereby increasing the risk of antibiotic resistance. To our knowledge, no study has yet explored the causal link and correlation between the presence of urinary tract anomalies and BMR UTI.

- In our series, a history of BMR infection confers a 12-fold risk of developing ESBL urinary tract infection similar to an American study by Dr Anesei et al which found that the presence of ESBL bacteria on a previous culture was an independent risk factor for ESBL infection (aOR, 12.75; P < 0.001) [29].

-There was no significant correlation between the severity of the urinary tract infection and germ resistance.

2.4 Characteristics of the infectious episode :

We recorded 37 cases of acute cystitis (60%) compared with 25 cases of PNA (40%), which is consistent with the literature. Cystitis was more frequent than pyelonephritis, with 56% cystitis compared with 43% pyelonephritis in the Tunisian series by Dr Ferjani et al, and 51.2% cystitis compared with 21.2% pyelonephritis in the series by Dr Essafi et al [30,31]. A ratio of 18 to 18 episodes of cystitis for 1 episode of pyelonephritis has been estimated [32].

2.4.1 Functional signs and physical examination :

• Cystitis :

In our study, the most frequent signs were urinary burning (32%), followed imperiosis (19%), urinary leakage (13%), pollakiuria (11%) and, less frequentlyhaematuria (8%). A normal clinical examination with an average temperature of 36.9°C was noted in all patients. The presence of signs bladder irritation in 48% of cystitis, mictional burning in 50% and pollakiuria in 42% were noted in the Tunisian series by Dr Rachdi et al, Hopital La Rabta[33] . Dr Kaim et al noted the presence of mictional burning as the most frequent sign with 38%, followed by dysuria with 5.7%, while pollakiuria was absent in an Algerian study dating from 2020 [34]. According to studies of patients with cystitis, the presence of dysuria in association with urgency, even in the absence of vaginal discharge and signs bladder irritation, is 90% predictive of acute cystitis [35].

• NAP :

The most frequent clinical sign was lumbar pain (48%), followed by suprapubic pain and digestive disorders in 12% of our cohort. A fever was observed in 28% of cases, while sensitivity to lumbar shaking was noted in 32% of cases. Dr Rachdi's study found lumbar pain in 6/50, digestive signs in 6/50 and general signs in 13/50 [33]. The Sfax study by Dr Ben Jemaa showed low back pain in 80% of cases, abdominal pain in 17.6%, digestive signs in 35% and fever in 72% of cases[36]. In a Moroccan series, at the Ibn Rochd University Hospital in Casablanca, carried out by Dr Bourquia, lumbar pain was noted in 41% of cases, pelvic pain in 3%, digestive problems in 21% and fever in 34%[37].

2.4.2 Imaging:

• Cystitis: In our cohort, 10 ultrasound scans were performed in patients with diabetes or renal failure who were normal. According to the SPILF 2017 recommendations, there is no indication imaging during simple acute cystitis. It is recommended if urinary retention is suspected or in cases of recurrent cystitis [38, 39,40].

• ANP: Ultrasound is only recommended for simple ANP if there is an unfavourable evolution after 3 days. A uroscanner or, failing that, an ultrasound scan is recommended for ANP at risk of complication (SPILF 2017) [38,39]. However, some studies recommend ultrasound or even a uroscanner for all cases of ANP [40].

2.4.3 Biology :

• Cystitis: Our series proves the uselessness of blood tests when the CBC and inflammatory markers are normal. Blood tests are not recommended during cystitis according to HAS- SPILF 2021 recommendations. Our series proves the uselessness of blood tests when the CBC and inflammatory markers are normal.

• ANP: Our series showed a predominantly neutrophilic hyperleukocytosis in 28% of cases. Leukopenia was noted in 12% with neutropenia and lymphopenia in 0.04% and thrombopenia in 12% of cases. This is explained by the presence of severe ANP: 3 cases of sepsis and 2 cases of septic shock. A CRP and renal work-up (+/- CBC) is recommended for all ANP at risk of complication according to HAS-SPILF 2021 recommendations. A systematic work-up is not recommended for all simple ANP [39].

2.4.4 Cytology :

Cystitis: Positive leucocyturia; defined as more than 1000 EB/ml or 10EB/mm3; in 91% of cases in our series. In the literature, leukocyturia has a reported sensitivity of 90% to 96% and a specificity of 47% to 50% when associated with urinary symptoms [42]. The absence of leucocyturia may exclude cystitis if the pre-test probability is low [43].

ANP: Leukocyturia was noted in 76% of patients with ANP and haematuria in 20% of cases. Leukocyturia was found in 77.5% of patients in a Korean series by Dr Song et al [19], who found a negative correlation between the absence of leukocyturia and previous antibiotic use, with a risk of 75.1%. Haematuria may be present in ANP, but other causes should be considered, such as urinary lithiasis or complications [45].

2.4.5 Culture :

BGN was isolated in 83.5% of patients. The most frequently isolated germ E. coli with 50.7% in our series against a prevalence between 62% and 71% in Tunisia and between 53 and 76% in North African countries (see table XXIV) followed by KP (20.9% against a prevalence according to series between 6.3% and 29.9%), Proteus mirabilis and gram positive Cocci. The most common micro-organisms in UTIs E. coli (50%), followed by KP and then other BGNs in a French series by Dr Lafforest et al [57]. In the Dr Savoye-Rossignol series, E. coli was the leading cause with 83%, followed by Proteus mirabilis with 4% and KP with 2.1% [58]. Similarly, a series of 26 French laboratories showed that E. coli was the most frequent germ (72%), followed by KP (9.75%), Proteus mirabilis (5.8%) and Enterobacter cloacae (2.9%), which is similar to our series [59].

Table XXIV shows the different germs isolated from studies carried out in North African countries.

Table XXIV: Bacteriological profile of urinary tract infections according to studies

Germs / Authors	E coli (%)	KP (%)	Proteus mirabilis (%)	Enterobacter (%) / E. cloacae(%)	Other BGN(%)	Enterococcus (%)	E. faecalis (%)	S. Saprophiticus (%)
Larabi [46] Tunis 1996-1998	69,5	9,3	4,7	-/ 2,2	2,8	-	1,3	4,9
Toumi [47] 2009-2013 Monastir	56,7	29,9	4,47	-/ 4,47	4,47	-	-	-
Ben Jmaa [36] Sfax 2012	61	20	2,2	3 / -	Pseudomonas=2 ,2	-	0,8	0,4
Aouf [48] Algiers 2010-2012	66,15	11,96	5,42	2,08/ -	-	-	-	-
Guermazi-Toumi [49] South of the tunisia 2015-2016	62	10,9	2,63	2,6/ 0,33	-	-	-	-
Mohamed [50] Libya 2016	55,6	16,3	6,3	-/ 2,5	Pseudomonas=5,6	-	-	-
Ait mimoune [51] Algeria 2019	24,44	6,3	3,33	-	Pseudomonas: 5.92 Acinetobacter 0.74	1,48	-	1,11
Jaoua [52] Ben Arous 2012-2019	66,3	13,7	3,8	-/ 1,8%				
Hamamouchi	68	23	-	-	9	-	-	-

[53] Morocco 2018-2020								
Brahimi [54] Algeria 2018-2020	53	21	13	-	Pseudomo nas=5	3	-	5
Ben Ashur [55] Libya 2020	55,68	20,46	9,09	-	Pseudomo nas: 10.23	1,81		
Benmoumou [56] Algeria 2021	76	13	13	-	-	-	-	-
Our Tunisia 2014-2023 series	50,7	20,9	3	1,5/ 3	4,4	3	1,5	1,5

E. coli: Esherchia coli, KP: Klebsiella pneumoniae, BGN: gram-negative bacillus, E. feacalis: Enterococcus faecalis: S. saprophytucus: Staphylococcus saprophyticus

2.4.6 Antibiotic resistance :

In our cohort, we isolated a BMR in 27% and ESBL-secreting bacteria in 13%. The ESBL-secreting species were enterobacteria (E. coli followed by Klebsiella pneumoniae, other BGN). The epidemiology of beta-lactamase-secreting germs causing UTIs was dominated by enterobacteria, with E. coli accounting for 65.2% in a Tunisian series by Dr Bougossa et al, 62% in the series by Dr Marrakechi et al [60, 61], and ESBL-secreting bacteria 7% in the series by Dr Aouf et al and 10.5% in the study by Dr Hamamouchi. In the Algerian series (Dr Aouf et al) and the Moroccan series (Dr Hamamouchi), Klebsiella pneumoniae was the most common with 21.5% and 36.1%, followed by E. coli in 4.65% and 3.3%, unlike our series with E. coli (37.5%) followed by Klebsiella pneumoniae (25%) [48,53].

The most frequent multi-resistance association was betalactam resistance with FQ at 94% (N=16), followed by betalactam resistance with sulfametoxazole-trimetroprime at 52.9% (N=9), then betalactam resistance with cyclines at 29.4% (N=8). The association between betalactam resistance and aminoglycosides was 17.6% (N=3). A Moroccan study by Dr Benaissa et al found a lower rate of co-resistance of betalactamins with FQs in 79% but a higher rate of co-resistance of betalactamins and sulphametoxazole-trimetroprime in 65% [62].

2.4.6.1 E. coli resistance profile

Penicillin

Escherichia coli during urinary tract infections are resistant to penicillins in 65.7% of cases, with values comparable to those observed in the Tunisian series by Jaoua et al (2012-2019) with 66% but lower than those of Ben Jemaa et al with 74% [36,52]. In Algeria, penicillin resistance was higher at 76% (Benmoumou series) but comparable to that of Aouf et al (66%) [48,56]. The values described in the Ben Ashur (Libya) study and the Farfour (France) study were lower at 38.7% and 50.9% respectively [55,59].

<u>Cephalosporin :</u>

Resistance to C3G was 6%, surpassing that of Dr Rachdi et al 2014 (4.5%), Aouf et al (Algeria) (5.6%) and Savoye-Rossignol et al (France) (1.5%) [33, 48,58]. However, it remains comparable to that of Farfour et al (France) (6.4%), Hamamouchi et al (Morocco) (6%) and Ben Jemaa (Sfax) (11.4%) [36,53,59].

<u>Fluoroquinolone :</u>

The rate of FQ resistance in Tunisia increased from 0.3% in 2002 (Laarbi et al) to 19.2% in 2012 (Ben Jmaa et al) and 29.4% (our series) in 2023 [36,46]. It is lower at 17.7% in northern Algeria (Aouf et al) and 2023% in Morocco (Hamamouchi et al) [48,53]. In France, resistance ranges from 1.5 to 13.1% depending on the series [58,59].

<u>Cotrimoxazole :</u>

Cotrimoxazole resistance (20.6%) has decreased compared with 2002 (Larabi et al: 46.9%) and 2019 (Jaoua et al: 35.15%) in Tunisia [46, 52]. This resistance is lower than that described in the series by Hamamouch et al (37.6%) and Ben Ashur et al (28.5%) [53, 55].

<u>Aminoside :</u>

A decrease in resistance rates from 14.6% in 2016 in the series by Guermezi et al to 6% in 2023 [49] has been observed. This resistance is similar to that of the Algerian study by Aouf et al (6.39) but lower than that of the Moroccan study by Bouamri et al (14%) [48,63].

<u>Fosfomycin and Nitrofurantoin :</u>

In our study, strains of E. coli resistant to Fosfomycin and Nitrofurantoin were identified. However, other studies have documented resistance ranging from 8.7% in Algeria (Aouf et al), 11% in Morocco (Bouamri et al) to 61% in Libya (Ben Ashur et al) to Nitrofurantoin [48,55,63].

Resistance to Fosfomycin was 0.19% in Tunisia in 2019 (Jaoua et al) and 0.5% in the series by Aouf et al (Algeria) [48,52].

■=> Our series showed a lower rate of resistance to penicillins (64.7% versus 72.9%), C3G (6% versus 17.3%), aminoglycosides (6% versus 11.2%), and Cotrimoxazole (20.6% versus 38.7%) compared to those observed by LART 2019. However, these strains showed a higher rate of resistance than FQ (29.4% versus 24.4%).

Table XXV summarises the main antibiotic resistances of E.coli.

Table XXV: Table summarising antibiotic resistance in Escherichia coli as a function of time and regions

Study	Bouamri Morocco	Rachdi Rabta	Guermazi Gafsa	Jaoua B.Arous	B.Ashur Libya	Benmoum or Algeria	Our Tunisi e

	2013 [63]	2014 [33]	2016[26] [49]	2019 [52]	2020 [55]	2021 [56]	2023 study
Amoxicillin	65%	68 %	78%	68,9%	38,7%	71%	64,7%
Amox-Ac clav	43%	38,6%	48%	29%	28,5%		57%
C3G	-	68%	11,9%	7,2%	44,9%	3-8%	6%
FQ	22%	59%	24,3%	-	57,14	7-9%	29,4%
Aminosides	8-14%	-	14,6%	8,3%	-	0	6%
Cotrimoxazole	55%	50%	46,6%	35,15	-	22%	20,6%
Fosfomycin	7%	-	-	0,19%	-	0	0%
Nitrofurantoine	11%	-	-	7,7%	61,22%	1%	0%

FQ: Fluoroquinolone- C3G: [3rd] generation cephalosporin- Amox-Ac clav: Amoxicillin-clavulanic acid

2.4.6.2 Resistance profile of Klebsiella pneumoniae

Penicillin :

The resistance of Klebsiella pneumoniae species isolated in our study is 57% to Amoxicillin-Clavulanic acid. This represents an increase compared with the 2016 cpmme described by Guermazi et al (38.9%) and the 2019 in Jaoua's series (29%) [49,52]. Resistance to Amox-ac clav is lower at 38.5% (Mohamed et al) in Libya, 32.7% in Morocco (Hamamouchi et al) and 28% in France (Farfour et al) [53,64, 59].

Fluoroquinolone :

Resistance to FQs was estimated at 16.7% in 2016 (Guermazi et al), decreasing to 14.3% in 2023 (our series) [49]. This rate is lower than that of Aouf et al (Algeria: 17.72%), Farfour et al (France: 17.9%) and Hamamouchi et al (Morocco: 25-31%) [48, 53, 59].

[3rd] generation cephalosporins:

No resistance to C3Gs was detected in our study whereas it reached rates of 38.5% in Libya (Mohamed et al) and 23% in Algeria (Aouf et al) [48, 54]. In France, the rate is 6.5% (Farfour et al) [59].

Aminoside :

Depending on the study, resistance to aminoglycosides varies between 10% as described by Hamamouchi et al (Morocco), 12.5% in Libya (Mohamed et al), 20.6% in the Algerian series by Aouf et al and 52% in the study by Ben Jemaa (Tunisia), but nil in this study [36,48,53, 64].

Cotrimoxazole :

Resistance to cotrimoxazole was 38% in 2016 in our country (Guermazi et al). This rate is nil in our study. It is high at 26.9% in Libya (Mohamed et al) and 23.4% in France (Farfour et al), but low at 7% in the Benmoumou series (Algeria) [49,56,59, 64].

■=> A comparison with the 2019 LART shows an increase in penicillin resistance (57.2% versus 43.7%), and a decrease in fluoroquinolone resistance

(14.3% versus 31.3%).

Table XXVI summarises the different values of resistance of Klebsiella pneumoniae to antibiotics according to the studies.

Table XXVI: Summary table of Klebsiella pneumoniae resistance according to different studies.

Studies	Aouf Algeria 2012	Mohamed Libya 2016	Guermazi Tunisia 2016	Jaoua Ben Arous	Benmoumou Algeria	Our Tunisia series
				2019		2023
Amox-Ac clav	34,27%	38,5%	38,9%	29%	11%	57,2%
C3G	23%	38,5%	25,35%	9,9%	1-3%	0%
FQ	23,9%	30,8%	16,7%	-	-	14,3%
Cotrimoxazole	37%	26,9%	38,46%	-	7%	0%
Aminoside	20,66%	53,8%	15,7%	7,8%	0	0%

Amox-Ac clav: Amoxicillin-clavulanic acid, C3G: 3rd generation cephalosporin, FQ: Fluoroquinolone

2.5 Prescribing antibiotics :

2.5.1 Empirical antibiotic therapy

a/ Cystitis

In the cystitis group, antibiotics were prescribed in 97.2% of cases. The majority were administered orally, with intravenous antibiotics being used in 13.5% of cases. The family of antibiotics most frequently prescribed empirically was FQ (32.4%), followed by C3G (29.7%) and Fosfomycin (3rd)) (16.2%). Cotrimoxazole was in 4th position with 5.4% followed by imipenem in last position (2.7%). Our results are comparable to those of Dr Essafi et al, who collected 330 prescriptions from 76 general practitioners. This study found that FQ was prescribed in 46.5% of cases of cystitis, while Fosfomycin and C3G were prescribed in 16% of cases and Nitrofurantoine in 5.2% [31]. In Algeria, the most frequently prescribed TBAs are cephalosporins and FQs [48].

A comparison with the prescription described in the study by Vorkaufer, which described the management of urinary tract infections in 66 doctors in Lorraine (France), showed that FQs were used in a similar proportion to our study (37%), followed by Nitrofurantoines (30%) and C3Gs (26%), in 3rd (as opposed to 2nd) position in the Tunisian studies[65].

FQs, which are not recommended either by the STPI 2018 or by the HAS-SPILF 2021, are prescribed first in Tunisia and France despite a high rate of resistance. A systematic review concluded that prescribing behaviour is a complex process based on internal and external factors [66]. Among these, the dominant perception of the prescriber is that patients want antibiotics and the fear of the consequences of not using ATBs [31,66]. The use of FQ is an example of the high rates of inappropriate prescribing associated with the treatment's availability, efficacy and broad spectrum of activity [31,67].

C3Gs are the 2nd [eiI1st] antibiotic prescribed in our cohort, compared with a low prescription rate of 5% in France, with resistance rates of 5.4% for germs and 11% for E. coli in our study. It is not one of the families recommended by the STPI and SPILF for cystitis. This high rate of prescription explains why the intravenous route is used in the majority of cases. A review of the therapeutic approach used in this cohort revealed that the clinical features that led to confusion between cystitis and ANP, the refusal of the oral route by some patients, and the often limited availability of treatments within the hospital were the arguments that justified this approach in our series.

Fosfomycin was prescribed in [3rd] position in our cohort, supported by Tunisian and French recommendations for simple acute cystitis at risk of complication, with a low resistance rate of 2.7%.

Cotrimoxazole, also known as trimethoprim-sulfamethoxazole, is prescribed at 5.4%. According to the STPI 2018, it is only indicated as a [2nd] choice for cystitis at risk of complication, but is not included in the HAS-SPILF 2021 recommendations.

Although Pivmecillinam is recommended in the treatment of uncomplicated cystitis by STPI 2018 and HAS-SPILF 2021, it was not prescribed in our cohort and is rarely prescribed in France.

Nitrofurantoin was also not prescribed in our cohort, despite the recommendations of the STPI 2018, which suggest it as the [first-line] treatment, and the absence of resistance in cystitis germs, probably explained by the low exposure of germs to this antibiotic. We note that it is recommended by the HAS-SPILF 2021 for acute cystitis at risk of complication.

■=> This therapeutic attitude towards 1st [ere] line prescribing during cystitis is not as consistent with recommendations. Despite its therapeutic efficacy, there is a risk worsening antibiotic resistance in Tunisia.

b/ NAP

In the ANP group, antibiotics were prescribed in 92% of cases. Most were administered intravenously in 82% of cases. Bitherapy was necessary in 20% of cases. The family of antibiotics most frequently prescribed empirically was C3G in 68% of cases, followed by FQ in 20% and then Aminosides in [3rd] position at 1.2%. Amoxicillin-clavulanic acid, imipenem and metronidazole were prescribed equally (0.4% each). The mean duration antibiotic treatment was 11.7 days (6-31 days).

This prescription pattern is similar to that described in the study by Ben Jmaa and Rachdi al: C3G was the most frequently prescribed antibiotic in 77.3%-60% of cases, followed by FQ (18.4%-52%) and aminoglycosides (17.5%) [33,36]. 40.8% of patients prescribed bitherapy, more than in our cohort (20%)[36].

In comparison with the therapeutic attitude described by Vorkaufer (in France), FQs are the most frequently prescribed antibiotics (63%), whereas C3Gs are prescribed in only 9% of cases [65].

C3Gs are recommended in 1st place by the STPI 2018 and in 2(nd) place by the HAS-SPILF 2021 for simple or severe acute pyelonephritis. Whereas FQs are only recommended by the STPI 2018 as a 3rd choice if simple ANP versus a 1st choice if simple ANP or risk of complication as a 1st choice if no FQ is taken within 6 months by the HAS-SPILF 2021. The study by Essafi et al found low adherence to recommendations (20.7%) for the management of UTIs in Tunisia in 2019, similar to that reported in France in 2011 [31].

Aminoside was prescribed at a rate of 1.2%, always in combination with other antibiotics (C3G), and is only recommended in combination with C3G as a first-line treatment or in combination with imipenem if severe NIP with ESBL risk factors, but as a 2nd second choice monotherapy if NIP at risk of complication without signs of severity, according to STPI 2018.

Imipenem is only indicated if there are risk factors for ESBL, which was the case in our cohort.

The STPI 2018 and HAS-SPILF 2021 do not recommend amoxicillin-clavulanic acid and metronidazole as first-line treatment for PNA. However, it was prescribed in 0.4% of cases.

A systematic review by Teixeira Rodrigues et al concluded that prescribing behaviour is a complex process based on a range of internal and external factors [31,66]. Among these, the prescriber's dominant perception is that patients want antibiotics and the fear of what might happen if antibiotics are not available [31,66]. FQ use is an example of the high rates of inappropriate prescribing associated with the treatment's availability, efficacy and broad spectrum of activity [67].

2.5.2 Treatment after antibiotic susceptibility testing

In the cystitis group, one case required escalation to cephalosporin. This can be explained by the resistance profile and the lack of availability of large quantities of antibiotics. Therapeutic de-escalation was possible after antibiotic susceptibility testing, but again was limited by the variable availability of the vast majority of treatments within the hospital.

In the ANP group, we had to escalate therapy in 2 cases. The antibiogram revealed 8% of ESBL germs (i.e. 2 germs) which were treated with Imipenem+ aminoside as recommended by STPI 2018. A switch to FQs was possible on the basis of the antibiogram.

This highlights the importance of re-evaluating and adapting empirical antibiotic therapy. However, the 48-72 hour delay in introducing effective antibiotics is a challenge in the management of infectious diseases. On the one hand, any delay, even within the hour, has an impact on infection-related mortality (septic shock) and, on the other, the consequences of a broad-spectrum antibiotic treatment on the individual's microbiota and the phenomenon antibiotic resistance. It is therefore necessary to develop "rapid" resistance detection techniques (detection of proteins, genes or enzymes involved in resistance) [68].

2.5.3 Relay processing

In the ANP group, a relay treatment was indicated in 20% of cases. It was indicated with the aim of switching to the oral route. This value is lower than that of the Ben Jmaa series, which described oral relay in 79.5% of cases.

Switching to the oral route reduces the length and cost of hospitalisation and complications associated with the access (venitis or nosocomial infection), and improves patient comfort. The oral route should therefore be considered as soon as possible [69].

2.5.4 Treatment duration

In the cystitis group, the average duration was 5 days, comparable to the durations indicated by STPI 2018.

The average duration of antibiotic treatment in the PNA group was 12 days, with a minimum of 6 days and a maximum of 31 days. This duration was insufficient in the minimum arm and too long for the maximum arm, given that the minimum indication for parenteral betalactamine was 7 days and the maximum 14 days according to STPI 2018, bearing in mind none of the patients received aminoglycoside as monotherapy. The duration of antibiotic therapy was shorter than that reported by Dr Ben Jmaa, with an average duration of 20 days (8-105), explained by the development of complications such as renal abscess or phlegmon [36], and that of Rachdi, which was 2.5 weeks (2-3 weeks) [33,36].

Recent studies have shown a tendency to shorten the duration of antibiotics. In the case urinary tract infections, some studies have shown that there is no inferiority between short and long courses [70, 71]. However, other studies have shown an inferiority of 7 days versus 14 days, particularly in terms of early recurrence [72].

In conclusion, there is a significant discrepancy between antibiotic prescriptions and those recommended by learned societies (STPI 2018 and HAS-SPILF 2021). This disparity is explained on the one hand by the local bacterial ecology and its resistance, and on the other hand by the non-availability of antibiotics in

Tunisian hospitals, their accessibility and their cost. In addition, the latest assessment of bacterial ecology and antibiotic resistance in Tunisia, the world's 2nd largest consumer antibiotics, dates from 2019. The study by Essafi et al has shown an increase in the inappropriate use of antibiotics in the Arab population, including Tunisia.

Self-medication, easy access to antibiotics and recourse to healthcare personnel other than the doctor is one of the major causes blamed for the increase in antibiotic resistance [31]. Several players are implicated:

- Patients and the general population have insufficient knowledge of antibiotics. They wrongly believe, for example, that ATBs can be used for viral diseases (influenza, fatigue, headaches). This to self-medication [73]. Another phenomenon reported by the general public is early discontinuation of antibiotic therapy as soon as the disease starts to improve [31]. Insufficient duration of antibiotic treatment is one of the main causes of resistance to ATBs.

- As Aboud et al [74] have shown, the accessibility and ease with which antibiotics can be obtained have a negative impact on drug uptake ( ).

- Healthcare professionals, led by doctors, prescribe the treatment without providing sufficient advice on how to take the ATB or monitoring the dose at a distance [31, 75].

Of course, non-compliance with national recommendations, dictated by the unavailability and high cost of treatments in hospitals and outpatient clinics alike, is accelerating this phenomenon, which is still preventable.

The lack of access to an expert (infectiologist), especially in clinics or in the city, can increase the risk prescribing errors in cases of confusion or doubt. This is confirmed by the work of Dr Bellazreg et al, who found that the intervention of the mobile antibiotic therapy team reduced the prescription of broad-spectrum ATBs from 61% to 50%, and the prescription of C3Gs from 22% to 15% [76].

We propose to carry out a multicentre, prospective study, recruiting care facilities in the interior and especially primary care physicians, in order to better identify and evaluate the daily practices of physicians as well as bacterial ecology resistance, especially after development of the national programme to combat antimicrobial resistance in Tunisia from 2019-2023.

On a national scale:

-Once the national programme to combat antibiotic resistance has been drawn up, ongoing monitoring tools will need to be developed, such a system for reporting anonymous antibiotic susceptibility test results from public and private laboratories.

-Develop a national alert system for regions where resistance exceeds an indicated threshold, in order to set up a control strategy adapted to the specific characteristics of the region.

-Establish a therapeutic strategy that takes account of the country's needs and the economic status of patients, and review it periodically.

-Require a medical prescription before selling any ATB.

<u>On the scale of healthcare professionals:</u>

-Physicians other than infectious diseases specialists, especially those practising in the private sector, need to have their knowledge and skills reinforced through annual courses and electronic media.

-Doctors need to be made more aware of the need to tailor their treatment to the sensitivity of the germs and the specific characteristics of the patient and the region in which they practise.

Other healthcare staff - nurses, orderlies, pharmacists and others - must be made aware of the need to stop prescribing antibiotics and issuing them without a doctor's prescription.

-He insisted on compliance with hygiene measures in all health and public facilities.

-It is important to explain how to take and monitor TBAs.

<u>On a population scale:</u>

The general public needs to be made aware of the harmful effects of self-medication or taking antibiotics without a prescription.

-I suggest developing advertising spots, newspapers and even brochures detailing these effects.

-Patients must be taught not to miss doses and to stick to the doses and duration prescribed by the doctor.

-The general public must be made aware of the need to avoid requiring healthcare professionals to administer antibiotics for every symptom.

-Inform patients about the therapeutic recommendations for urinary tract infections, the signs of improvement and worsening, and the need therapeutic adherence.

6 Conclusion

Urinary tract infection is the second most common community infection after respiratory tract infection. This frequent pathology affects women in particular.

Urinary tract infection is still a topical issue, especially in view of the increasingly alarming level of antibiotic resistance in a country ranked as the world's 2nd largest consumer antibiotics.

The main aim of our study was to describe the therapeutic management of UTIs in women outside pregnancy in an internal medicine department.

We conducted a retrospective, descriptive, monocentric study of the records of patients hospitalized for UTI in the Internal Medicine Department of the Razi Hospital in Tunis between January 2016 and August 2023.

Sixty-two non-pregnant patients were included with an average age of 59 years. Diabetes and hypertension were the most frequent pathological antecedents. 19% of patients had a BMR FDR. The patients had cystitis in 60% of cases and PNA in 40%. Burning micturition was present in 32%, dysuria in 30% and pollakiuria in 13%. Macroscopic haematuria was present in 8%. Patients reported fever in 25% and back pain in 24%.

SIB was present in 96% of ANPs and PNN hyperleukocytosis was present in 28% of ANPs. ARF was present in 44% of ANPs.

Leukocyturia was present in a comparable manner between PNA (92%) and cystitis (91%). Microscopic haematuria was present in 20% of cases of ANP and 5.4% of cystitis. Culture was negative in 8% of ANPs and 13% of cystitis. Enterobacteriaceae were the most frequent germs. The most common E. coli with 56% in both cystitis and PNA, followed by KP with 25% in cystitis and 17% in PNA. BMR were present in 27% and secreted ESBL bacteria in 13%. The most frequently isolated BMR E. coli, followed by KP. E.coli was penicillin-resistant in 64.7%, FQ-resistant in 29.4% and ESBL-secreting in 8.8%. KP was resistant to Amox-Ac clav in 57.2%, to FQ in 14.3% and secreted ESBL in 14.3%. In the ANP group, the most commonly prescribed antibiotic was C3G in 68%, followed by FQ in 20%. Bitherapy was required in 20%. Oral relay was prescribed in 20%. The mean duration of antibiotic treatment was 12 days (6-31 days).

In the cystitis group, FQs were the most frequently prescribed antibiotics (32.4%), followed by C3Gs (29.7%). The mean duration was 5 days (1-7 days).

Recent studies have shown a trend towards shortening the duration of antibiotics.

Analytical analysis showed that there was a statistically significant relationship between diabetic nephropathy and BMR urinary tract infection, between urinary tract abnormalities and ESBL infection, and between hypertension and FQ resistance. A history BMR infection increased the risk of developing ESBL urinary tract infection by 12-fold. was also no relationship between the severity of urinary tract infection and BMR infection.

Non-compliance with national recommendations, dictated by the unavailability and high cost of treatments in hospitals and outpatient clinics alike, is accelerating antibiotic resistance, even though it is still preventable.

Self-medication, easy access to antibiotics, recourse to healthcare personnel other than the doctor and early cessation of antibiotic therapy are among the major causes blamed for the worsening of antibiotic resistance.

Recommendations for the correct use of antibiotics must be applied at patient, doctor and national level in order to antibiotic resistance.

7 References

1.   Schmiemann, G., Kniehl, E., Gebhardt, K., Matejczyk, M. M. & Hummers-Pradier, E. The diagnosis of urinary tract infection: a systematic review. Dtsch. Arzteblatt Int. 107, 361 (2010)

2.   Hickling DR, Sun TT, Wu XR. Anatomy and Physiology of the Urinary Tract: Relation to Host Defense and Microbial Infection. Microbiol Spectr. 2015 Aug;3(4):10.1128/microbiolspec.UTI-0016-2012.

3.   Mlugu, E.M., Mohamedi, J.A., Sangeda, R.Z. *et al.* Prevalence of urinary tract infection and antimicrobial resistance patterns of uropathogens with biofilm forming capacity.

4.   Nicolle LE. Uncomplicated urinary tract infection in adults including uncomplicated pyelonephritis. Urol Clin North Am. 2008 Feb;35(1):1-12, v.

5.   Foxman B, Barlow R, D'Arcy H, et al. Urinary tract infection: self-reported incidence and associated costs. Ann Epidemiol 2000;10:509-15.

6.   Rowe TA, Juthani-Mehta M. Diagnosis and management of urinary tract infection in older adults. Infect Dis Clin North Am. 2014 Mar;28(1):75-89.

7.   Ben Redjeb. S, Boutiba-Ben Boubaker. I, Saidani. M, Antibiotic resistance in Tunisia, LART Data 20082010 - Edition July 2013

8.   Klein EY, Van Boeckel TP, Martinez EM, Pant S, Gandra S, Levin SA, Goossens H, Laxminarayan R. Global increase and geographic convergence in antibiotic consumption between 2000 and 2015. Proc Natl Acad Sci U S A. 2018 Apr 10;115(15):E3463-E3470.

9.   Lee CR, Cho IH, Jeong BC, Lee SH. Strategies to minimize antibiotic resistance. Int J Environ Res Public Health. 2013 Sep 12;10(9):4274-305.

10.   https://www.has-sante.fr/upload/docs/application/pdf/2021-11/dossier_press_release_antibioresistance.pdf ANTIBIORESISTANCE: From research to action, all mobilised to antibiotic resistance: HAS

11.   Yang X, Chen H, Zheng Y, Qu S, Wang H, Yi F. Disease burden and long-term trends of urinary tract infections: A worldwide report. Front Public Health. 2022 Jul 27;10:888205. doi: 10.3389/fpubh.2022.888205. PMID: 35968451; PMCID: PMC9363895.

12.   Naber K.G., Tiran-Saucedo J., Wagenlehner F.M.E. Psychosocial burden of recurrent uncomplicated urinary tract infections. *GMS Infect. Dis.* 2022;10:Doc01. doi: 10.3205/id000078.

13.   Grigoryan L., Mulgirigama A., Powell M., Schmiemann G. The emotional impact of urinary tract infections in women: A qualitative analysis. *BMC Women's Health.* 2022;22:182. doi: 10.1186/s12905-022-01757-3.

14.   Harrington R.D., Hooton T.M. Urinary tract infection risk factors and gender. *J. Gend.-Specif. Med. JGSM Off. J. Partnersh. Women's Health Columbia.* 2000;3:27-34. [PubMed] [Google Scholar]

15.   Andolfi C., Bloodworth J.C., Papachristos A., Sweis R.F. The Urinary Microbiome and Bladder Cancer: Susceptibility and Immune Responsiveness. *Bladder Cancer* 2020;6:225-235. doi: 10.3233/BLC- 200277. [PMC free article] [PubMed] [CrossRef] [Google Scholar]15)

16.   Gdoura S, Dridi K, Profil des infections urinaires communautaires a germes producteurs de beta lactamases a   spectre   elargi,   La   STPI   et   la   SPILF,   sep   2021.   Available   at   URL: https://www.infectiologie.org.tn/uplcadEposter/4514.pdf

17.   Lahlou Amine I, Chegri M, L'Kassmi H. Epidemiology and antibiotic resistance of enterobacteria isolated from urinary tract infections at the Moulay-Ismail military hospital in Meknes. Antibiotiques. 2009 May;11:90-96.

18.   Guibert J, Destree D, l'Infection urinaire du sujet age revue generale - Traitement par le ciprofloxacine- Medecine et Maladies Infectieuses - MAI 1988 : 33 -336

19.   Benoit T, Leguevaque P, Roumiguie M , Beauval J.B. , Malavauda B, Soulie M. , et al, ffistrogenotherapie locale   en   urologie   et   pelvi-perineologie.   Revue   de   litterature,   jan   2015.   Available   at https://doi.org/10.1016/j.purol.2015.01.012

20.   Ballager P, Epidemiology of urinary incontinence in women Progres en Urologie (2005), 15, Supp. N°1, 1322-1333

21.   Kumar S, Muchmore A. Tamm-Horsfall protein--uromodulin (1950-1990). Kidney Int. 1990 Jun;37(6):1395- 401. doi: 10.1038/ki.1990.128. PMID: 2194064.

22.   BARRIER LETERTRE C, URINARY INFECTIONS IN THE ELDERLY: difficulties in microbiological diagnosis and the impact of prescribing ECBU for the management of the elderly at Angers University Hospital [These: pharmacy]. Angers University; 2014

23.   El Aziz, S.; Haraj, N.; Hassoune, S.; Obbiba, A.; Chadli, A.; El Mdaghri, N.; El Ghomari, H.; Farouqi, A.

(2014). *Prevalence and factors associated with urinary tract infection in diabetic women at the Casablanca University Hospital Centre, Morocco. Medicine of Metabolic Diseases, 8(2),   204 210.* doi:10.1016/S1957-2557(14)70742-4

24. Andy I.M. Hoepelman; Ruby Meiland; Suzanne E. Geerlings (2003). *Pathogenesis and management of bacterial urinary tract infections in adult patients with diabetes mellitus. ,   22(supp-S2),   35 43.* doi:10.1016/s0924-8579(03)00234-6

25. Affes L, Mnif F, Cheikhrouhou N, Hadjkacem F, Charfi N, Abid M, Urinary tract infections and diabetes: a propos de 100 cas, Service d'endocrinologie et diabetologie, CHU Hedi Chaker, Sfax, Tunisie, 2016 . Available at: https://doi.org/10.1016/j.ando.2016.07.782

26. Saada L, Kooli I,* Kadri Y, Abdejlil M, Marrakchi W, Aouam A, et al , Les bacteries multiresistantes (BMR) chez le diabetique : etude epidemio-clinique , SFE Marseille 2020 / Annales d'Endocrinologie 81 (2020) 408-456 Available at https://www. em-consulte.com/article/1393242/les-bacteries-multiresistant-bmr-chez-le-diabeti

27. chakroun H , Rouis S, Ben Lasfar N, Abid M, Bellazreg F, Hachfi W, Letaief A? Evolution de la prevalence et les facteurs de risque des infections a BMR dans le service de Maladies Infectieuses de Sousse, STPI et SPILF, sep 2021 consultable sur https://www.infectiologie.org.tn/uploadEposter/4044.pdf

28. Kalla N, Ouanassa H, Noui L, Melizi A, Aouidane S, Merzougui Z, Les facteurs de risque d'acquisition des infections a BMR,Algerie, LA TUNISIE MEDICALE - 2024 ; Vol 102 (n°03)

29. Anesi JA, Lautenbach E, Tamma PD, Thom KA, Blumberg EA, Alby K, Bilker WB, Werzen A, Tolomeo P, Omorogbe J, Pineles L, Han JH. Risk Factors for Extended-Spectrum в-lactamase-Producing Enterobacterales Bloodstream Infection Among Solid-Organ Transplant Recipients. Clin Infect Dis. 2021 Mar 15;72(6):953- 960. doi: 10.1093/cid/ciaa190. PMID: 32149327; PMCID: PMC7958726.

30. Ferjani S; Saidani M; Ennigrou S; Hsairi M; Ben Redjeb S (2012). *Virulence determinants, phylogenetic groups and fluoroquinolone resistance in Escherichia coli isolated from cystitis and pyelonephritis, 60(5), - .* doi:10.1016/j.patbio.2011.07.006

31. Essafi S, Omezzine Letaief A, Phillips E, Vardanega V, Antimicrobial stewardship and economic evaluation of urinary tract infection management in primary health care in Tunisia, Family Medicine & Primary Care Review 2021; 23(3): 295-300

32. Li R, Leslie SW. Cystitis. [Updated 2023 May 30]. In: StatPearls [Internet]. Treasure Island (FL): StatPearls Publishing; 2024 Jan-. Available from: https://www.ncbi.nlm.nih.gov/books/NBK482435/

33. Rachdi I, Ben Ghorbel I, Khanfir M, Hamzaoui A, Ben Salem T, Said F, Lamloum M, et al, Clinical manifestations and treatment of urinary tract infections: A comparative study according to the age, al ,La Rabta Hospital, Tunisia, Late Breaker Posters / European Geriatric Medicine 5S1 (2014) S235-S253

34. KAIM N, KOUACHE H, Le profil clinique et bacteriologique de l'infection urinaire (Memoire, microbiologie] Canstantine, Universite des Freres Mentouri Constantine, 2020

35. Bent S, Nallamothu BK,_ Simel DL; Fihn S D ; Saint S , This Woman Have an Acute Uncomplicated Urinary Tract Infection? JAMA. 2002;287(20):2701-2710. doi:10.1001/jama.287.20.2701

36. BEN JMAA M, ACUTE PYELONEPHRITIS IN DIABETICS. ETUDE DE 348 CAS. [thesis, infectiology] Sfax, Faculte de Medecine de Sfax

37. BOURQUIA A, Sahni K, Zaid D, RAMDANI B, PROFILE OF URINARY INFECTION IN A NEPHROLOGY DEPARTMENT. Medecine du Maghreb 1992 n°33

38. Diagnosis and antibiotic therapy of community-acquired bacterial urinary tract infections in adults. Recommandations de la Societe de Pathologie Infectieuse de Langue Fran^aise (spilf) 2017.

39. Community urinary tract infections: Cystitis, pyelonephritis and male urinary tract infection- HAS-SPILF-recommendation 2021, Updated 19 May 2023,

40. Bjerklund J. The role of imaging in urinary tract infections. World J Urol 22, 392-398 (2004). https://doi.org/10.1007/s00345-004-0414-z

41. Diagnosis and antibiotic therapy of bacterial urinary tract infections   infections in adults. Recommandations de la Societe de Pathologie Infectieuse de Langue Fran^aise (spilf) 2015.

42. Lala V, Leslie SW, Minter DA. Acute cystitis. [Updated 2023 Jul 10]. In: StatPearls [Internet]. Treasure Island (FL): StatPearls Publishing; Jan 2024-. Available at: https://www.ncbi.nlm.nih.gov/books/NBK459322/

43. Stephen T. Chambers, Sarah C. Metcalf, Cystitis and Urethral Syndromes, in Infectious Diseases (Fourth Edition), 2017,

44. Song HK, Shin DH, Na JU, Han SK, Choi PC, Lee JH. Clinical investigation on acute pyelonephritis without pyuria: a retrospective observational study. J Yeungnam Med Sci. 2022   Jan;39(1):39-45. doi:

10.12701/yujm.2021.01207. Epub 2021 Aug 11. PMID: 34411474; PMCID: PMC8895969.

45. Belyayeva M, Jeong JM. Acute pyelonephritis. [Updated 2022 Sep 18]. In: StatPearls [Internet]. Treasure Island (FL): StatPearls Publishing; 2024 Jan-. Available from: https://www.ncbi.nlm.nih.gov/books/NBK519537/

46. Larabi [K], Masmoudi K, Fendri C, Etude bacteriologique et phenotypes de résistance des germes responsables d'infections urinaires dans un CHU de Tunis : a propos de 1930 cas, Medecine et Maladies Infectieuses, Volume 33, Issue 7, July 2003, Pages 348-352

47. Toumi A , Aouam A, Ben Brahim H, Marmouch H, Loussaief C , Chakroun M, Profil bacteriologique des infections urinaires chez les sujets diabetiques , Annales d'Endocrinologie Vol75-N 5-6, P398 oct 2014

48. Aouf A , Gueddi T , Djeghout B , Ammari H, Frequency and susceptibility pattern of uropathogenic Enterobacteriaceae isolated from patients in Algiers, Algeria , J Infect Dev Ctries 2018; 12(4):244-249. doi:10.3855/jidc.1001

49. Guermazi-Toumi S, Boujlel S, Assoudi M, Issaoui R, Tlili S, Hlaiem ME. Susceptibility profiles of bacteria causing urinary tract infections in Southern Tunisia. J Glob Antimicrob Resist. 2018 Mar;12:48-52. doi: 10.1016/j.jgar.2017.09.004. Epub 2017 Sep 14. PMID: 28918351.

50. Mohammed MA, Alnour TS, Shakurfo OM, Aburass MM, Prevalence and antimicrobial resistance pattern of bacterial strains isolated from patients with urinary tract infection in Messalata Central Hospital, Libya, Asian Pacific Journal of Tropical Medicine, Volume 9, Issue 8,2016,Pages 771-776,Available at (https://www.sciencedirect.com/science/article/pii/S1995764516301286)

51. Ait-Mimoune N, Hassaine H, Boulanoir M. Bacteriological profile of urinary tract infections and antibiotic susceptibility of Escherichia coli in Algeria. Iran J Microbiol. 2022 Apr;14(2):156-160. doi: 10.18502/ijm.v14i2.9180. PMID: 35765552; PMCID: PMC9168253.

52. Jaoua MA, Dhraief S, Frigui S, Oueslati M, Krir A, Thabet L, Epidemiologie et evolution de la résistance aux antibiotiques des germes uropathogenes communautaires dans la région de Ben Arous , 30eme Congres National de la STPI et 1er Congres Francophone de Pathologie Infectieuse et de Microbiologie Clinique, Cahier des resume 2021, p 385 , sep 2021

53. Hamamouchi J, Qasmaoui A , Halout K , Charof R, Ohmani F , Antibiotic resistance in uropathogenic enterobacteria , E3S Web of Conferences 319, 01 (2021) VIGISAN 2021

54. Brahimi H, Bousselhem A, Douahi O, Benshouk S, Profil de résistance des bacilles a gram negatif uropathogenes isoles au CHU Telmcen , 30eme Congres National de la STPI et 1er Congres Francophone de Pathologie Infectieuse et de Microbiologie Clinique, Cahier des resume 2021, p 385 , sep 2021

55. Ben Ashur A ,El Magrahi H, Elkammoshi A, Alsharif H ,Prevalence and Antibiotics Susceptibility Pattern of Urine Bacterial Isolates from Tripoli Medical Center (TMC), Tripoli, Libya ,IBEROAMERICAN JOURNAL OF MEDICINE 03 (2021) 221-226

56. Benmoumou S, Hamaidi-Chergui F, Bouznada K , Bouras N, Bakli M and Meklat A, Antibiotic Resistance Pattern of Enterobacteriaceae Strains Isolated from Community Urinary Tract Infections in Algiers, Algeria, ADVANCED RESEARCH IN LIFE SCIENCES Jul, 2023, p46 - 53

57. De Lafforest S, Magnier A, Vallee M, Le Goux C, Zahar J, Sotto A, Bruyere F, Grammatico-Guillon L, Incidence des infections urinaires hospitalisees en France : une cohorte historique, Infectious Diseases Now 51 (2021) S103-S106,Volume 51, Issue 5, Supplement, 2021,Pages S103-S104, Borquiahttps://doi.org/10.1016/j.idnow.2021.06.214 .,(https://www.sciencedirect.com/science/article/pii/S2669991921003304)

58. Louise Savoye-Rossignol. Epidemiology of community-acquired urinary tract infections. Public health and epidemiology. Universite Pierre et Marie Curie - Paris VI, 2015. Fran^ais. ffNNT: 2015PA066378ff. fftel-01275795f

59. Farfour E, Dortet L, Guillard T, Chatelain N, Poisson A, Mizrahi A, et al On Behalf Of The Gmc Study Group. Antimicrobial Resistance in Enterobacterales Recovered from Urinary Tract Infections in France. Pathogens. 2022 Mar 15;11(3):356.

60. Bougossa R, Marrakchi W, Kooli I, Ben Brahim H, Loussaief C, Toumi A, et al les infections urinaires a enterobacteries secretrices des beta-lactamases a spectre elargi dans un service de medecine, 30eme Congres National de la STPI et 1er Congres Francophone de Pathologie Infectieuse et de Microbiologie Clinique, Cahier des resume 2021, p 385 , sep 2021

61. Marrakchi W, Aouam A, Kooli I, Kadri Y, Ben Brahim H, Loussaief C, et al ,Les infections urinaires communautaires a enterobacteries secretrices de в-lactamase a etendu spectre chez les sujets diabetiques : what are the particularities? Service des Maladies Infectieuses CHU F. Bourguiba Monastir. SFE Congress 2016

,Available at https://www.congres-sfe.com/2016/eposters/60993588-7265-11e6-9efb-d97ff2406a52.pdf

62. Benaissa E, Belouad E, Mechal Y, Benlahlou Y, Chadli M, Maleb A, Elouennass M. Multidrug-resistant community-acquired urinary tract infections in a northern region of Morocco: epidemiology and risk factors. Germs. 2021 Dec 29;11(4):562-569. doi: 10.18683/germs.2021.1291. PMID: 35096673; PMCID: PMC8789347.

63. El Bouamri MC, Arsalane L, Kamouni Y, Yahyaoui H, Bennouar N, Berraha M, Zouhair S. Current antibiotic resistance profile of uropathogenic Escherichia coli strains and therapeutic consequences. Prog Urol. 2014 Dec;24(16):1058-62. French. doi: 10.1016/j.purol.2014.09.035. Epub 2014 Oct 11. PMID: 25310915.

64. Mohammed MA, Alnour T, Shakurfo O, Aburass M, Prevalence and antimicrobial resistance pattern of bacterial strains isolated from patients with urinary tract infection in Messalata Central Hospital, Libya,Asian Pacific Journal of Tropical Medicine,Volume 9, Issue 8,2016,Pages 771 776.https://www.sciencedirect.com/science/article/pii/S1995764516301286)

65. Vorkaufer S. Community-acquired bacterial urinary tract infections in adults: diagnostic and therapeutic management. Results of two rounds of a clinical audit carried out by 66 general practitioners in Lorraine. Sciences du Vivant [q-bio]. 2011. ffhal-01733536, [These, medecine genarale],

66. Teixeira Rodrigues A, Roque F, Falcao A, et al. Understanding physician antibiotic prescribing behaviour: a systematic review of qualitative studies. Int J Antimicrob Agents 2013; 41: 203-212

67. Aldred KJ, Kerns RJ, Osheroff N. Mechanism of quinolone action and resistance. Biochemistry 2014; 53: 1565-1574.

68. Decousser JW, Pozzetto B, Romano-Bertrand S. L'antibiogramme: techniques rapides et tests complementaires. Hygienes 2023;31(4):331-337.

69. McCarthy K, Avent M. Oral or intravenous antibiotics? Aust Prescr. 2020 Apr;43(2):45-48. doi: 10.18773/austprescr.2020.008. Epub 2020 Apr 1. PMID: 32346210; PMCID: PMC7186270.

70. Lee RA, Stripling JT, Spellberg B, Centor RM. Short-course antibiotics for common infections: what do we know and where do we go from here? Clin Microbiol Infect. 2023 Feb;29(2):150-159. doi: 10.1016/j.cmi.2022.08.024. Epub 2022 Sep 6. PMID: 36075498.

71. McAteer J, Lee JH, Cosgrove SE, Dzintars K, Fiawoo S, Heil EL, Kendall RE, Louie T, Malani AN, Nori P, Percival KM, Tamma PD. Defining the Optimal Duration of Therapy for Hospitalized Patients With Complicated Urinary Tract Infections and Associated Bacteremia. Clin Infect Dis. 2023 May 3;76(9):1604-1612. doi: 10.1093/cid/ciad009. PMID: 36633559; PMCID: PMC10411929.

72. Lafaurie M, Chevret S, Fontaine JP, Mongiat-Artus P, de Lastours V, Escaut L, Jaureguiberry S, Bernard L, Bruyere F, Gatey C, Abgrall S, Ferreyra M, Aumaitre H, Aparicio C, Garrait V, Meyssonnier V, Bourgarit-Durand A, Chabrol A, Piet E, Talarmin JP, Morrier M, Canoui E, Charlier C, Etienne M, Pacanowski J, Grall N, Desseaux K, Empana-Barat F, Madeleine I, Bercot B, Molina JM, Lefort A; PROSTASHORT Study Group. Antimicrobial for 7 or 14 Days for Febrile Urinary Tract Infection in Men: A Multicenter Noninferiority Double-Blind, Placebo-Controlled, Randomized Clinical Trial. Clin Infect Dis. 2023 Jun 16;76(12):2154- 2162. doi: 10.1093/cid/ciad070. PMID: 36785526.

73. Abduelkarem AR, Othman AM, Abuelkhair ZM et al. Prevalence of self-medication with antibiotics among residents in United Arab Emirates. Infect Drug Resist 2019; 12: 3445-53. https://doi. org/10.2147/IDR.S224720

74. Abood EA, Scott J, Wazaify M. User experiences of prescription and over-the-counter drug abuse in Aden City, Yemen. Pharmacy 2018; 6: 99.https://doi.org/10.3390/pharmacy6030099

75. Ali M, Abbasi BH, Ahmad N et al. Over-the-counter medicines in Pakistan: misuse and overuse. Lancet 2020; 395: 116116. https:// doi.org/10.1016/s0140-6736(19)32999-x

76. Bellazreg F, Ben Lasfar N, Abid M, Rouis S, Hachfi W, Letaief A. Antibiotic stewardship team in a Tunisian university hospital: A four-year experience. Tunis Med. 2022 May;100(5):403-409. PMID: 36206090; PMCID: PMC9552246.

STPI 2018

Cystites simples

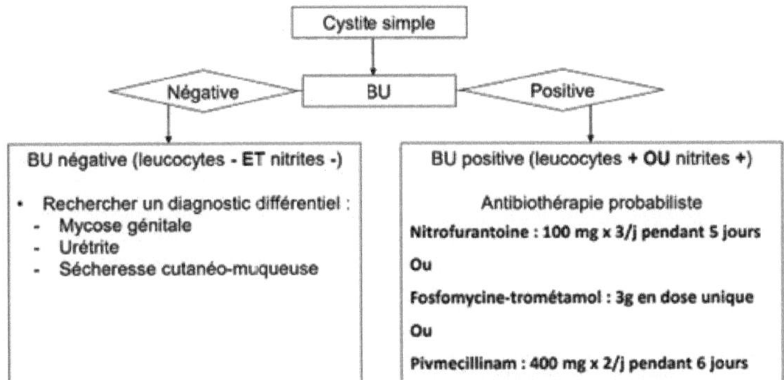

Cystites à risque de complication

PNA sans signe de gravité
Traitement initial probabiliste

PNA simple :

- C3G parentérale : céfotaxime ou ceftriaxone *[A-1]*

ou

- Aminoside, en l'absence de FDR de néphrotoxicité :

      gentamicine ou amikacine *[B-2]*

ou

- FQ, si 1ᵉʳ épisode et en dehors des FDR de résistance aux FQs: ciprofloxacine ou ofloxacine *[A-1]*

PNA à risque de complication :

- C3G parentérale : céfotaxime ou ceftriaxone *[A-1]*

ou

- Aminoside, en l'absence de FDR de néphrotoxicité :

      amikacine ou gentamicine *[C-4]*

Facteurs de risque de néphrotoxicité des aminosides
. **Age avancé** (> 75 ans)
. Utilisation concomitante **d'autres médicaments néphrotoxiques ou de produits de contraste iodés**
. **Déshydratation**
. **Insuffisance rénale** (clairance de la créatinine < 60 ml/min)
. **Néphropathie** préexistante ou concomitante
. **Cirrhose sévère** de grades B et C selon la classification de Child-Pugh
. Prise de **médicaments favorisant l'hypoperfusion** rénale (diurétiques de l'anse, inhibiteurs de l'enzyme de conversion ou antagonistes de l'angiotensine II, anti-inflammatoires non stéroïdiens)

Facteurs de risque de résistance aux FQs : prise de FQs ou hospitalisation dans les 6 mois précédents

PNA grave
Traitement initial probabiliste

céfotaxime ou ceftriaxone + amikacine *[C-4]*

Sauf dans les cas suivants :

- Sepsis ou nécessité de drainage (avec ATCDs de colonisation ou d'infection urinaire à BLSE dans les 6 mois):

      Imipénème + Amikacine *[A-1]*

- Choc septique avec ≥ 1 facteur de risque de BLSE:

      Imipénème + Amikacine

En cas d'allergie aux C3G ou aux carbapénèmes :

      Amikacine + Fosfomycine *[accord professionnel]*

    ou Amikacine + Colimycine *[accord professionnel]*

Cystite aiguë simple

Symptômes de la cystite: brûlures mictionnelles, pollakiurie, impériosité/urgenturie ou dysurie dits signes fonctionnels urinaires (SFU), urines troubles ou hématuriques.

Prise en charge de la cystite par BU (leucocytes+ voire nitrites+) et antibiothérapie probabiliste.

1. **Fosfomycine trométamol**
   https://base-donnees-publique.medicaments.gouv.fr/affichageDoc.php?specid=66430643&typedoc=R
   3g dose unique
2. **Pivmécillinam**
   https://base-donnees-publique.medicaments.gouv.fr/affichageDoc.php?specid=60670489&typedoc=R
   (Selexid®) 400 mg x 2/j pendant 3 jours

ECBU uniquement en l'absence d'amélioration à 72 heures, récidive dans les 2 semaines ou double contre-indication. Le traitement adapté à l'antibiogramme sera celui des cystites à risque de complication.

Traitement « minute » possible chez la jeune fille uniquement si pubère (*SPILF 2020*).

En cas de BU négative, rechercher un diagnostic différentiel: mycose, urétrite, sécheresse cutanéo-muqueuse.
Une BU peut être réalisée en pharmacie avec orientation vers le médecin en cas de positivité.

En cas de cystite aiguë sur sonde urinaire: 3 jours d'antibiothérapie (*SPILF 2020*)

Cystite aiguë à risque de complication

ECBU en cas de facteur de risque de complication ① et antibiothérapie différée autant que possible.

Antibiothérapie probabiliste uniquement en cas de symptômes marqués:

1. **Nitrofurantoïne**
   https://base-donnees-publique.medicaments.gouv.fr/affichageDoc.php?specid=62013296&typedoc=R
   (Furadantine®) 100 mg x 3/j pendant 7 jours
   Sauf clairance < 45 mL/min.
2. Fosfomycine trométamol 3g dose unique

Antibiotique de préférence adapté à l'antibiogramme:

1. Amoxicilline 1g x 3/j pendant 7 jours
2. Pivmécillinam (Selexid®) 400 mg x 2/j pendant 7 jours
3. Nitrofurantoïne 100 mg x 3/j pendant 7 jours

ECBU de contrôle uniquement en l'absence d'amélioration à 72 heures ou récidive précoce dans les 2 semaines.

Bladder-scan si suspicion de rétention aiguë d'urines.

Pyélonéphrite aiguë simple

Antibiothérapie probabiliste juste après l'ECBU:

1. **Ciprofloxacine 500 mg x 2/j ou lévofloxacine 500 mg/j**
   Sauf fluoroquinolone dans les 6 mois.
2. Ceftriaxone IM 1 g/j (2g si obèse)
3. Hospitalisation

Échographie rénale sous 24 heures si évolution défavorable après 72 heures d'antibiothérapie

Adaptation à l'antibiogramme dès le rendu des résultats:

1. **Amoxicilline 1g x 3/j pendant 10 jours**
2. Cotrimoxazole 800/160 mg x 2/j pendant 10 jours
3. Amoxicilline-acide clavulanique 1g x 3/j pendant 10 jours
4. Ciprofloxacine 500 mg x 2/j ou lévofloxacine 500 mg/j ou ofloxacine 200 mg x 2/j pendant 7 jours
5. Céfixime 200 mg x 2/j pendant 10 jours
6. Ceftriaxone IM 1 g/j pendant 7 jours (2g si obèse)
7. Entérobactérie productrice d'E-BLSE
   a. Ciprofloxacine ou lévofloxacine ou cotrimoxazole
   b. Amoxicilline-acide clavulanique
   c. Céfoxitine
   d. Hospitalisation

Réévaluation systématique à 72 heures.
ECBU de contrôle uniquement en cas d'évolution défavorable après 72 heures.

Pyélonéphrite aiguë à risque de complication

En présence d'une pyélonéphrite avec facteur de risque de complication ① sans signe de gravité:

- Bilan biologique: CRP, créatininémie
- Uroscanner en urgence (max 24h) ou à défaut échographie rénale

Antibiotiques identiques à la pyélonéphrite aiguë simple (chapitre précédent) pendant 10 jours.

Réévaluation systématique à 72 heures.
ECBU de contrôle uniquement en cas d'évolution défavorable après 72 heures.

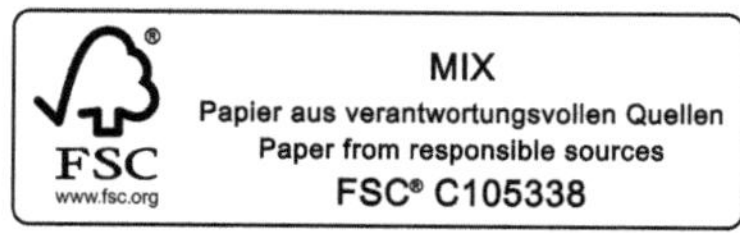

Printed by Books on Demand GmbH, Norderstedt / Germany